AJPH
A PUBLICATION OF THE
AMERICAN PUBLIC HEALTH ASSOCIATION

AMERICAN JOURNAL of PUBLIC HEALTH
MARCH 2026
Issue 3

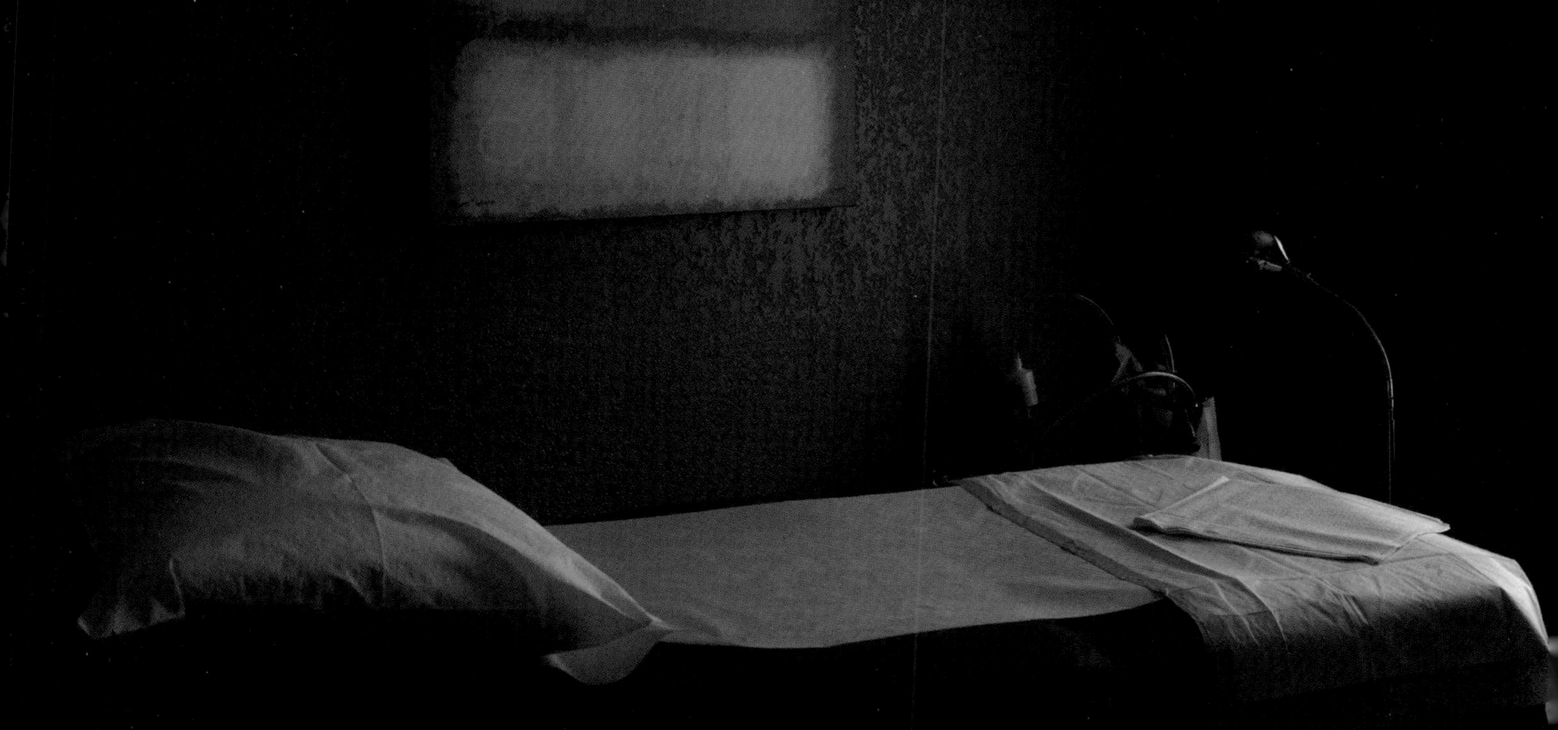

Abortion and Public Health in Post-*Dobbs* Era

- Reframe Reproductive Autonomy
- Trust in Maternal Health Data
- Maternal and Infant Health
- Impact on States Without Bans

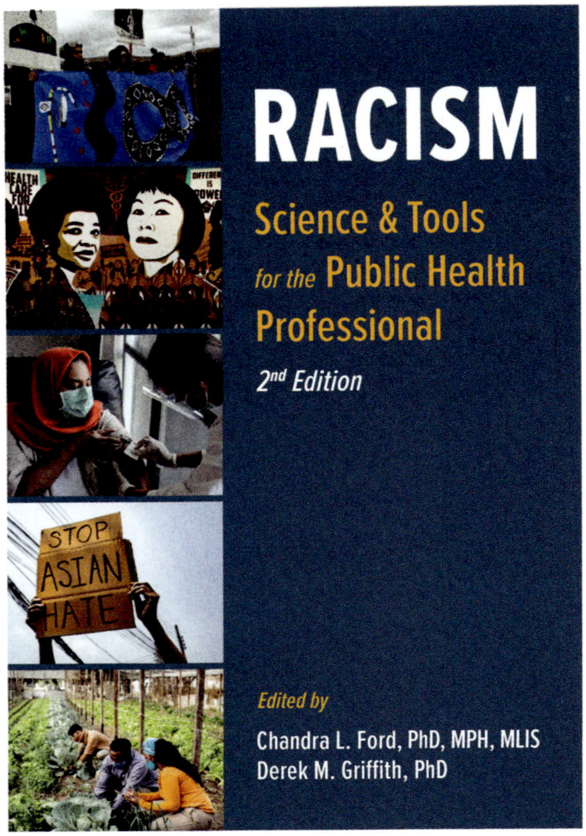

Racism: Science and Tools for the Public Health Professional, 2nd edition

Chandra L. Ford, PhD, MPH, MLIS, and Derek M. Griffith, PhD

ISBN 978-0-87553-352-0, 600 PP., 2025, SOFTCOVER

Racism: Science and Tools for the Public Health Professional, 2nd edition enables public health professionals to address the health impacts of racism. This vital title also responds to the watershed events of the past five years: the COVID-19 pandemic and its intersection with overt forms of racism across all socioecological levels, the 2020 murder of George Floyd by Minneapolis police and the unprecedented domestic and global movements toward racial justice that transpired, and other major global events.

APHA
AMERICAN PUBLIC HEALTH ASSOCIATION
For science. For action. For health.

AJPH®, published monthly, is the official Journal of the American Public Health Association®, 800 I St NW, Washington, DC 20001-3710; (202) 777- APHA; TDD (202) 777-2500. APHA is a nongovernmental professional society founded in 1872, representing all disciplines and specialties in public health.

The *American Journal of Public Health*® (*AJPH*) (print ISSN: 0090-0036; electronic ISSN: 1541-0048), first published in 1911, is the official journal of the American Public Health Association® (APHA). The oldest and largest organization of public health professionals in the world, APHA represents approximately 30 000 members from more than 50 occupations of public health.

Submissions: Visit www.editorialmanager.com/ajph for online manuscript preparation and submission guidelines. Contributions of original unpublished research, social science analyses, scholarly essays, critical commentaries, departments, and letters to the editor are welcome. Questions? Write ajph.submissions@apha.org or call APHA at (202) 777-2469.

Print plus online subscriptions: Institutional price (print copy with online access) for a single institution and all authorized users, regardless of geographic location varies by size of organization; multiple campuses not permitted without special arrangement. To order, write apha.subscriptions@apha.org.

Online-only subscriptions: Institutional price for one US federal institution and its authorized users is $1,015–$1,510. To order, write apha.subscriptions@apha.org. For academic, non-US federal consortia, or multisite subscriptions, contact apha.subscriptions@apha.org or visit http://research.ebsco.com for pricing information.

Print-only subscriptions: Institutional price is US $970, $1,065 international.

Back print issues: A limited number of print issues are for sale. Single copies are US $80, $90 international (air delivery). Shipping and handling fees will apply; prepay only. To order, write apha.subscriptions@apha.org.

Reprints: For prices and ordering information on 50 or more reprints, check the Reprints section at www.ajph.org. To order smaller quantities of reprints (rush delivery), use the "Purchase Article" link on the article site itself.

Electronic access: Online articles more than 10 years old are available free for personal use at www.ajph.org. Recent articles are available through pay-per-view: single PDF article for $24, single issue access for 24 hours for $33, or entire site access for 24 hours for $38.

Postal information: Periodicals postage paid at Washington, DC, and additional mailing offices. Postmaster: Send address changes to American Journal of Public Health, 800 I St NW, Washington, DC 20001-3710.

Address changes: Send to AJPH, Membership Department (members) or AJPH Subscriptions (subscribers), APHA, 800 I St NW, Washington, DC 20001-3710. Or write to membership.mail@apha.org (members) or apha.subscriptions@apha.org (subscribers).

Advertising: For pricing and other information, see www.ajph.org. Please write to brian.selzer@apha.org or call (202) 777-2464 for other advertising opportunities. Ask about special exhibit packages and sponsorships. Acceptance of advertising by the *Journal* does not imply endorsement of products.

Indexes: Publications that index or abstract articles from *AJPH* include the following: Ageline, Assia (Applied Social Science Index and Abstracts), Biological Abstracts, Chemical Abstracts, CINAHL, Criminal Justice Abstracts, EMBASE, EMCare, Environmental Abstracts, e-psyche, ERIC, ETOH (Alcohol and Alcohol Problems Science Database), Excerpta Medica, Food Science and Technology, General Science Index, Grateful Med, Hospital Literature Index, Human Resources Abstracts, International Pharmaceutical Abstracts (IPA), Medline, Physical Education Index, Pollution Abstracts, Psychological Abstracts, PsychINFO, Safety Science Abstracts, Sage Family Studies Abstracts, Sage Human Resources Abstracts, Science Citation Index, SCOPUS, SIIC Data Bases, Social Work Research and Abstracts, and Statistical Reference Index (SRI)/LexisNexis.

Medscape Publishers' Circle

AJPH

A PUBLICATION OF THE
AMERICAN PUBLIC HEALTH ASSOCIATION

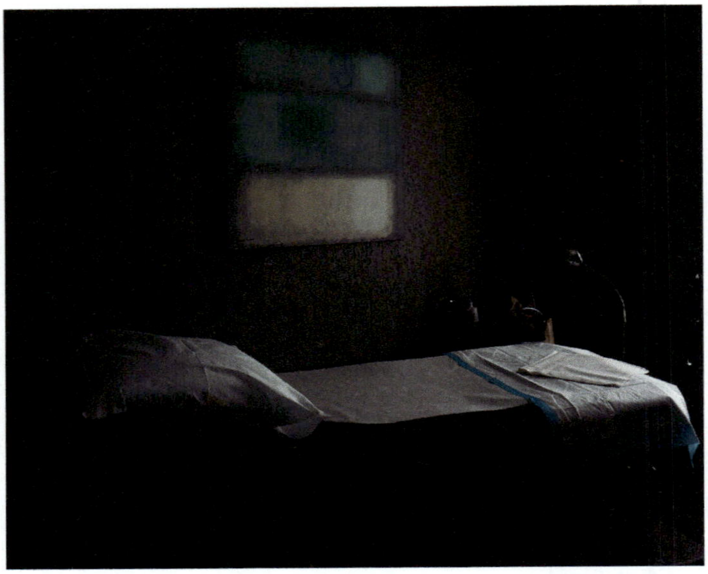

COVER: An examination room is empty at Wyoming's last abortion clinic, Wellspring Center, on March 10, 2025, in Casper, Wyoming. In late February, Wyoming's conservative legislature passed bill HB42, requiring abortion clinics performing in-clinic procedures to meet the regulatory requirements of ambulatory surgical centers, causing the clinic to pause all services.

Cover concept and image selection by Aleisha Kropf. Photo by Natalie Behring/Getty Images. Printed with permission.

APHA
AMERICAN PUBLIC HEALTH ASSOCIATION
For science. For action. For health.

Promoting public health research, policy, practice, and education is the *AJPH* mission. As we widen our scope to embrace global issues, we also sharpen our focus to support the needs of public health practitioners. We invite contributions of original unpublished research, opinion and commentary, and letters to the editor.

The *Journal* is printed on acid-free recycled paper.

OPEN ACCESS ONLINE ONLY PODCAST DATA SUPPLEMENT AVAILABLE

EDITOR'S CHOICE

284 A Risk We Cannot Afford: Public Health Must Be Recognized as a Professional Degree
L. Magaña

OPINIONS, PRACTICE, & EDUCATION

EDITORIALS FROM THE ACADEMICS

286 Working Across Sectors and Political Lines to Consider Health in All Policy Decisions
K. M. Pollack Porter

VACCINE ACCESS

289 Public Health Controversies: *AJPH*'s Series on Public Health Transformation and Vaccines
B. O. Ojikutu and D. T. Lau

292 Filling the Federal Void Through Shared Leadership in Vaccine Policy
D. M. Higgins

EDITORIALS

295 October 2025 Attempted Workforce Reduction Puts US Principal Health Statistics Agency at Risk
J. D. Schoendorf and D. T. Lau

298 Transgender and Gender-Diverse Rights and Health: A Global Perspective
M. C. Grinspan and S. Gruskin

300 Measure Racism, Not Just Race: Recommendations for Scientific Practice
F. T. Enders, P. M. Alberti, E. H. Golembiewski, M. A. Orellana, P. Braveman, V. A. Brown, N. Chambwe, C. L. Ford, and J. E. Balls-Berry

304 Evidentiary Pragmatism in Transgender Health Care
F. Ashley

NOTES FROM THE FIELD

307 A Venue-Based Approach to Asymptomatic Mpox Screening and Doxy-PEP Provision: From Outbreak to Outreach, San Francisco, California, 2023–2024
C. A. Contag, Z. T. Renfro, A. X. Mukund, M. Quint, S. Amitin, V. Levy, P. L. Hammack, B. A. Pinsky, and B. Laniakea

312 Umoja Health: Building Community Coalitions to Achieve Health Equity From COVID-19 to Cancer
K. F. Rhoads, E. N. Pardo, S. Ribeiro, G. Andemeskel, M. LeSarre, N. Aboelata, L. M. Tealer, D. Francis, Z. Harper, K. M. Mehta, J. D. Fuchs, and K. Watkins-Tartt

ABORTION AND PUBLIC HEALTH IMPACT IN POST-*DOBBS* ERA

317 Post-*Dobbs* Era: Evolving Abortion Care Restrictions and Public Health Impact
D. T. Lau, J. Liu, and M. M. Jones

321 Structural Violence and Reproductive Justice
A. E. Yamin

323 Post-*Dobbs* Realities: Ethical Imperatives for Data Transparency and Trust in Maternal Health Care
F. E. Fletcher, S. L. Schott, K. Akhiemokhali, and K. White

326 The Opportunity of Abortion-Protective States in the Post-*Dobbs* Era: Implications for Public Health Policy and Practice
S. K. Redd, S. Filippa, A. A. Luke, H. V. McMahon, and E. Chew Murphy

RESEARCH & ANALYSIS

ABORTION AND PUBLIC HEALTH IMPACT IN POST-*DOBBS* ERA

329 Reproductive Autonomy Restrictions as Collective Violence
N. J. Santaularia Gomez, K. Neumann, M. Tanveer, K. Farkas, and M. Altman

337 Changes in Facility-Based Abortion Care Among Texas Resident Minors and Young Adults After a 2021 Abortion Ban: September 2020–May 2022
K. White, G. Sierra, B. Whitfield, K. Tocce, S. L. Dickman, and V. Goyal

341 The Association Between State Gestational Age Limit Abortion Laws and Severe Maternal Morbidity: United States, 2010–2022
N. Siegal and A. Soni

345 Changes in Frequency and Health of Live Births Following State Abortion Bans
M. E. Wallace, Y. Wang, and C. Stoecker

351 Examining Post-*Dobbs* Changes in Abortion Use at 3 Southern Michigan Clinics, July 2021–June 2023
M. H. Smith, C. Sucher, A. Norris, V. K. Dalton, and S. D. Compton

359 Clinic Adaptations and Changes in Abortion Use After *Dobbs* in Illinois, July 2021–June 2023
M. H. Smith, D. Young, H. Dismer, V. Diskin, L. Hasselbacher, K. Rivlin, D. Bessett, and A. H. Norris

DATA & MONITORING

368 Validating Georgia's Vaccine Registry for the COVID-19 2023–2024 Season: True GRITS
A. D. Roebling, N. E. Barrera-Nitz, M. Tobin-D'Angelo, K. P. Openo, and L. S. Witt

OPEN-THEMED RESEARCH

372 Trends in Prepregnancy Cardiometabolic Health in Rural and Urban Areas in the United States, 2016–2023
H. Pedamallu, T. Nayak, A. A. Freedman, K. K. Venkatesh, W. A. Grobman, S. S. Khan, and N. A. Cameron

376 Estimated Number of People Who Inject Drugs in the United States, 2022
H. Bradley, S. N. Glick, and E. W. Hall

380 Racial Disparities in Victim Compensation Program Claim Approvals for Adult Survivors of Sexual Assault: 18 US States, 2015–2023
S. Dickman, J. Levine, C. Bolton, A. Conway, and K. Russell

387 Bridging the Hearing Divide: Policy Solutions for Aging Americans
M. R. Swamy, R. Marottoli, and A. B. Cohen

A Risk We Cannot Afford: Public Health Must Be Recognized as a Professional Degree

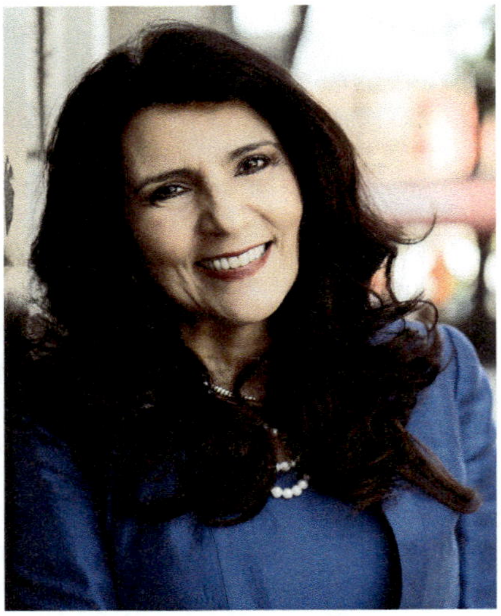

Laura Magaña, PhD, MS
President and CEO
Association of Schools and Programs of Public Health

The US Department of Education's Reimagining and Improving Student Education committee recently reached a preliminary consensus on a proposed narrower definition of "professional degree programs" under the One Big Beautiful Bill Act (Pub L No. 119–21 [2025]). The new definition by default excludes advanced degree public health programs as well as several other health profession programs. This recommendation is shortsighted and may have dangerous consequences. Excluding public health risks delaying—and, in some cases, completely stopping—the education and training of the next generation of practitioners and leaders responsible for protecting the nation's health.

I cannot speculate on why the federal government might want to dismantle the nation's public health infrastructure, but public health must remain nonpartisan.

Public health as a profession has a rich, more than a century-long history. In 1916, the Johns Hopkins School of Hygiene and Public Health, the world's first independent graduate school of public health, was founded. By 1936, there were 10 schools of public health in the United States. The Council on Education for Public Health, the primary US accrediting body for public health schools and programs, was established in 1974 to oversee the quality and standards of professional public health education; it defines a professional degree, such as MPH and DrPH, as a degree that prepares graduates for public health practice (https://bit.ly/4sq11mf).

Removing MPH and DrPH from the professional degree category after such a long history would immediately restrict students' access to federal loan resources, increase costs, and make these degrees less attainable for many. Degrees for nurses, physician assistants, social workers, physical therapists, and other essential health care professionals are also excluded. This proposal not only weakens the pipeline of future public health workers, researchers, and scientists but also disregards decades of precedent that recognize these degrees as vital professional credentials. If the department proceeds, these core degrees—proof that our frontline leaders are properly trained—will become very difficult, if not impossible, for many Americans to achieve. The impact would last for decades, harming the health and well-being of millions and undoing progress that has saved countless lives.

This is happening amid increasing threats to public health. Public health professionals protect and improve the health and quality of life for people and their communities. Their work is the backbone of community health, providing health education, disaster response, injury and disease prevention, environmental protections, and interventions for issues such as infant and maternal mortality, climate change, and the spread of infectious diseases.

Federal budgets are shrinking, experts are being dismissed, and state legislatures across the country are passing bills that weaken—or even undo—public health protections. A recent Associated Press investigation reviewed more than 1000 antiscience bills; more than 400 of these targeted proven measures, such as vaccines, milk safety, and water fluoridation (https://bit.ly/4jolRyi). Many states have already enacted these laws, creating a patchwork system of health protections that leaves communities vulnerable. We might not yet see the full impact of these decisions, but the consequences are inevitable. When they happen—whether the harm is physical, mental, or environmental—we will need highly trained public health professionals prepared to lead the response. That need is especially urgent now, with the workforce already shrinking and funding cuts speeding up.

During a time when chronic conditions and mental health issues are at historic highs and immunization rates keep dropping, our nation cannot afford to retreat. An Association of Schools and Programs of Public Health report released in June 2025 revealed that chronic disease now makes up 90% of US health care costs, even though half of these conditions are preventable (https://bit.ly/45Ga7l8). If we truly aim to reduce chronic disease and promote healthy longevity—ostensibly the goals of Make America Healthy Again—we need to strengthen, not weaken, our ability to train public health professionals.

Public health graduates are everywhere, working to keep us safe and healthy. They staff state and local health departments, hospitals, federal agencies, and community organizations. Public health workers provide vital support to rural communities, where residents often travel long distances for health care. The public health workforce also plays a key role in national security by monitoring outbreaks worldwide and preventing bioterrorism. They ensure that our food is safe, our water is drinkable, and our air is breathable. They study disease trends, develop innovative interventions to extend healthy lives, connect people with essential health resources, investigate environmental threats, analyze data to guide decisions, and offer policy advice. Unfortunately, ongoing cuts to the workforce and federal budget are forcing some public health departments to make difficult choices, such as cutting programs that fight obesity, provide prenatal care to reduce infant mortality, and prevent drug overdoses. Sadly, many health departments cannot do everything—and the nation will feel the consequences.

Some may argue that the nation's public health system needs a thorough overhaul. That may be true. However, making public health degrees more difficult to obtain—especially during a time of increased need and fewer resources—is not the solution. Millions will suffer if we prevent those who want to protect our communities from gaining the education they need. Public health practice is more than just a career; it is a calling. Those pursuing this profession deserve full support. Now is not the time to make earning a public health degree nearly impossible. Cancer, diabetes, heart disease, and mental illness do not care about political affiliation: they affect us all. Perhaps the effort is seen as a cost-cutting measure. Sicker Americans, an unsafe food supply, and unprepared states will not save us money, nor will they save lives. These policy changes could have the opposite effect: increasing our vulnerability to disease, undermining the foundations of healthy living, reducing our ability to recover from natural disasters, and widening health disparities. At a time when resilience is crucial, we cannot afford policies that set us back.

Congress must examine the Department of Education's proposal and the significant harm it could inflict on public health students, the workforce, and the nation's health. Congress can pass legislation to clarify that MPH, DrPH, and related degrees remain fully eligible for all federal support available for professional degrees. Lawmakers would benefit from reviewing the student impact data compiled by Association of Schools and Programs of Public Health member institutions, including forecasts on student debt, financial aid eligibility, enrollment, and workforce readiness.

The Department of Education is urged to update its proposed definition to include public health professional degrees and recognize them alongside other accredited professional programs. This is not just about academic titles or graduation ceremonies; it is about the health and safety of our families, communities, and nation. It is about ensuring that every American has the opportunity to live a long, healthy life and that well-trained public health professionals are ready to lead us into the future.

The health of the nation is at stake. That is worth standing up for. AJPH

DOI: https://doi.org/10.2105/AJPH.2025.308382

ORCID iD:
Laura Magaña https://orcid.org/0000-0002-6767-4339

Working Across Sectors and Political Lines to Consider Health in All Policy Decisions

Keshia M. Pollack Porter, PhD, MPH

ABOUT THE AUTHOR

Keshia M. Pollack Porter is the 12th dean of the Johns Hopkins Bloomberg School of Public Health, Baltimore, MD. She is also a Bloomberg Centennial Professor in the department of Health Policy and Management.

AJPH March 2026, Vol. 116, No. 3

Engaging across sectors has always been a part of my journey as a public health professional. As a doctoral student at the Johns Hopkins Bloomberg School of Public Health (BSPH), I studied injury prevention with Susan P. Baker, a founder of the field and one of my mentors. She taught me the importance of working with transportation professionals to design safer roads, architects and planners to design safer buildings and neighborhoods, employers to create safer workplaces, and manufacturers to design safer products. She underscored the significance of effectively engaging with others, especially those outside the health field who are making decisions that affect safety.

This approach spurred my interest in health impact assessment (HIA). HIAs rely on data and effective engagement with decision-makers from nonhealth sectors and the public to identify the potential positive and negative health implications of proposals and strategies to promote health and mitigate harms.[1] I believed in the power of HIAs to support policymaking and intersectoral partnerships, and it became a core part of my research, teaching, and practice.[2–4]

As dean of the BSPH and an expert in health policy, I continue to promote HIAs and other tools that advance Health in All Policies (HiAP).[5] This supports my vision to create a world where considering the potential health impacts of policy proposals is the norm. We know there are inextricable links between health and housing, transportation, education, and planning. The health impacts of all policies should be studied and shared with policymakers and the public to influence decisions—whether it's a proposal for paid parental leave, new roadways, or a local farm-to-school program.

MAKING THE CASE FOR ADOPTION OF HEALTH IN ALL POLICIES

HiAP has been implemented globally for decades in some jurisdictions, which provides important lessons about impacts and challenges.[6] Benefits of implementing HiAP include increased intersectoral collaboration, accountability of policymakers, and capacity across government agencies to integrate health into decision-making.[6–8] Challenges to advancing HiAP include lack of prioritization by policymakers, support for policy goals other than health, insufficient capacity and resources, and lack of systems-wide changes to sustain efforts.[6–8] Despite these challenges, I see tremendous opportunities to advance HiAP in the United States, especially at the local and state levels, and I offer three reasons why.

First, HiAP provides a framework to engage communities and policymakers. This involves authentically engaging communities that would be affected by the proposed policy, so they have power in the decision-making process. During a scoping workshop for a rapid HIA of a proposed redevelopment project in Baltimore, Maryland that I worked on, we asked residents how those proposed changes could affect health. They envisioned how redevelopment could reduce violence, increase access to food, and improve walkability. They also voiced concerns about how redevelopment could make it harder to afford housing, which could result in long-term residents being pushed out and the loss of community connections and cohesion. These critical insights highlighted the factors that needed to be addressed for community buy-in. We also engaged policymakers and other stakeholders to understand their goals and vision. This engagement helped build trust and ensure that health considerations from various groups were elevated as we made recommendations for how to both proceed with the project and promote health.

Second, flexibility and adaptability make HiAP viable for various contexts; there is no one way to "do" HiAP. For instance, HIAs are not always the best tool for policy decisions, especially ones that need to be made during short legislative sessions. With the support of colleagues whom I worked with at the Health Impact Project in Washington, DC, in 2017, I created a legislative health note, to ensure that legislators had a better understanding of how bills related to many sectors—from education to utilities—can affect health.[9] Inspired by fiscal notes, which elevate the potential fiscal impacts of bills, legislative health notes put health at the center of decision-making and fit the legislative context to achieve HiAP goals. Today, legislative health notes are conducted by the Health in All Policies Initiative at the BSPH, which I direct. We are teaching students at the BSPH about this tool and engaging with practitioners across the country to promote its utility. In fall 2025, our team completed a legislative health note for a ballot initiative in Colorado to increase taxes on high earners to fund universal free school meals.[10] The analysis showed the benefits of universal free school meals programs for all children: improved nutrition, reduced food insecurity, less financial strain for families, and reduced stigma and administrative burdens. This work was well-timed because an estimated 55 000 Coloradans stood to lose Supplemental Nutrition Assistance Program benefits because of federal changes, and the excess tax revenue could support the state's food assistance program.

The analysis was shared with local advocates and academic partners in Colorado to put the focus on health leading up to the elections. Early evaluation data from our implementation of legislative health notes found that they increased awareness of how nonhealth policies affect health,[9] and we bet that they could do the same in Colorado. On Election Day 2025, Colorado delivered a public health victory: more than 57% voted in favor of the tax increase.[11]

Third, HiAP values partnerships, which are essential to advance health. HiAP experiences worldwide reveal that HiAP works when the public health sector is listening and learning from other sectors, engaging with humility, and strengthening partnerships that create co-benefits. I acknowledge that engaging with other sectors is difficult. Policy and performance goals vary across sectors and may even be in conflict. Our work has revealed that creating ways for sectors to regularly assemble, communicate, identify common goals, and build trust can help to advance HiAP. We saw this in Maryland, when a statewide HiAP workgroup that included representatives from various sectors was established to strengthen intersectoral partnerships to identify co-benefits and advance health equity.[12]

CONCLUSIONS

Public health as a field is at a crossroads. Mistrust and misinformation about proven strategies to improve health, such as vaccines, are common. The federal government has rapidly changed the public health and research ecosystems, jolting how we operate. Moreover, health outcomes are not improving, health disparities are persistent or widening, and many communities are getting sicker and dying earlier.

We need a new way forward, and I believe that HiAP can help us get there. Advancing HiAP is possible even in challenging and divisive political environments. People of all political beliefs want to be healthy. And, to put it bluntly, health conditions don't know or care who you voted for in the last election. A HiAP approach can ensure that policies are health-promoting for everyone.

I don't believe my vision will be easy to achieve. I know that in some parts of this country, using words like public health or health equity can close doors. Moreover, I am not naïve enough to think that health can always be the primary consideration in policymaking. But I do believe that—through advocacy, communication, and engagement—we can increase the use of HiAP tools to ensure that health is routinely considered alongside factors like constituent demands and fiscal constraints. Through a HiAP framework, public health has an opportunity to show policymakers and the public just how practical and powerful our work can be. HiAP can help transform the systems that influence the drivers of health and health outcomes. By shaping policies that support health, we can reaffirm the value of public health and continue working toward a better and healthier future for everyone. AJPH

CORRESPONDENCE

Correspondence should be sent to Keshia M. Pollack Porter, 615 N. Wolfe St, Dean's Office, Baltimore, MD 21205 (e-mail: bsph.deansoffice@jhu.edu). Reprints can be ordered at https://www.ajph.org by clicking the "Reprints" link.

PUBLICATION INFORMATION

Full Citation: Pollack Porter KM. Working across sectors and political lines to consider Health in All Policy decisions. *Am J Public Health*. 2026;116(3): 286–288.

Acceptance Date: November 19, 2025.

DOI: https://doi.org/10.2105/AJPH.2025.308370

ORCID iD:

Keshia M. Pollack Porter https://orcid.org/0000-0001-5363-5462

ACKNOWLEDGMENTS

I thank members of the communications team at the Johns Hopkins Bloomberg School of Public Health for their review of the article.

Note. The perspectives in this article are the author's, and they are not representing the view or position of the Johns Hopkins University or Bloomberg School of Public Health.

CONFLICTS OF INTEREST

The author has no real or potential conflicts of interest to declare.

REFERENCES

1. National Research Council. *Improving Health in the United States: The Role of Health Impact Assessment.* Washington, DC: National Academies Press; 2011.
2. Pollack KM, Dannenberg AL, Botchwey N, Stone CL, Seto E. Developing a model curriculum for a university course in health impact assessment in the USA. *Impact Assessment and Project Appraisal.* 2015;33(1):80–85. https://doi.org/10.1080/14615517.2014.960213
3. Waimberg J, Cloud LK, Campbell AT, Lindberg R, Pollack Porter K. Tracking state-level health impact assessment legislation from 2012–2016. *CHIA.* 2018;3(1):1–10. https://journals.indianapolis.iu.edu/index.php/chia/article/view/22249
4. Sohn EK, Stein LJ, Wolpoff A, Lindberg R, Baum A, McInnis-Simoncelli A, Pollack KM. Avenues of influence: the relationship between health impact assessment and determinants of health and health equity. *J Urban Health.* 2018;95(5):754–764. https://doi.org/10.1007/s11524-018-0263-5
5. Rudolph L, Caplan J, Ben-Moshe K, Dillon L. *Health in All Policies: A Guide for State and Local Governments.* Washington, DC and Oakland, CA: American Public Health Association and Public Health Institute; 2013.
6. World Health Organization. Key learnings from health in all policies implementation from around the world. April 2018. Available at: http://www.who.int/publications/i/item/WHO-CED-PHE-SDH-18.1. Accessed November 11, 2025.
7. Shankardass K, Renahy E, Muntaner C, O'Campo P. Strengthening the implementation of health in all policies: a methodology for realist explanatory case studies. *Health Policy Plan.* 2015;30(4):462–473. https://doi.org/10.1093/heapol/czu021
8. Cain R, Greece JA, Galea S, et al. Improving health across sectors: best practices for the implementation of health in all policies approaches. *Prev Med Rep.* 2022;29:101961. https://doi.org/10.1016/j.pmedr.2022.101961
9. Carignan S, Lindberg R, Tung G, Sullivan J, Stone C, Pollack Porter KM. Legislative health notes: preliminary learnings from piloting a New Policy analysis tool. *J Public Health Manag Pract.* 2024;30(3):E135–E142. https://doi.org/10.1097/PHH.0000000000001866
10. Carignan S, Weston C. Legislative health note: Propositions LL and MM: Colorado Healthy School Meals for All. November 2025. Available at: https://publichealth.jhu.edu/sites/default/files/2025-10/CO-LL-MM-Legislative-Note-10.23.25-FINAL.pdf. Accessed November 12, 2025.
11. Dolven T. Colorado voters approve tax increase on high earners to fund school meals, food stamps. *The Colorado Sun.* Available at: https://coloradosun.com/2025/11/04/proposition-mm-results-colorado-election-2025. Accessed November 12, 2025.
12. University of Maryland School of Public Health Center for Health Equity. Senate Bill 340: University of Maryland School of Public Health Center for Health Equity—Workgroup on Health in All Policies. January 2018 report. Available at: https://msa.maryland.gov/megafile/msa/speccol/sc5300/sc5339/000113/023300/023335/20180471e.pdf. Accessed November 9, 2025.

Public Health Controversies: *AJPH's* Series on Public Health Transformation and Vaccines

Bisola O. Ojikutu, MD, MPH, and Denys T. Lau, PhD

ABOUT THE AUTHORS

Bisola O. Ojikutu is an AJPH *associate editor and is with the Boston Public Health Commission, Boston, MA, and Mass General Brigham, Boston, MA. Denys T. Lau is the editor-in-chief of* AJPH *and is with Johns Hopkins University, Bloomberg School of Public Health, Baltimore, MD, the Milken Institute of Public Health, George Washington University, Washington, DC, and the Retzky College of Pharmacy, University of Illinois, Chicago.*

See also Higgins et al., p. 292.

The US government's public health system is undergoing a profound transformation. Some might describe this directional shift as a strategic pivot designed to restore public trust, which has eroded since the COVID-19 pandemic. Others might characterize the shift as a misguided, disruptive, politically motivated deviation from our country's long-standing public health mission, scope, and fundamental values. Either way, many are confused and skeptical about this transformation because of the chaos and uncertainties these recent shifts have created.

Regardless of perspective, the changes that have occurred thus far at the federal level have been dramatic and unprecedented, including reducing the workforce, cutting funding, eliminating entire offices and work units, and ceasing engagement in the global public health ecosystem. Inarguably, nowhere has this transformation been more disturbing than in the directional shift of federal vaccination guidance that rebukes established scientific evidence in favor of debunked theories based on political ideologies. This transformation undoubtedly will have a significant impact on the health and well-being of communities across our nation.

More than 60 years ago, the Advisory Committee on Immunization Practices (ACIP) was established as a formal federal body composed of nongovernmental members. ACIP's objective was to provide independent expert guidance to federal public health decision-makers on the use of vaccines in the US civilian population.[1] In June 2025, the Trump administration disbanded the existing 17-member group and replaced its members with appointees, many of whom have previously expressed antivaccine sentiments.[2] In addition, influential professional organizations, such as the American Academy of Pediatrics and the American Medical Association, were removed from ACIP workgroups. Since its establishment, the newly configured ACIP has questioned the safety and efficacy of selected vaccines, discredited published research, and suggested several changes to the vaccine schedule.

The most notable recent change shifts from recommending universal birth dose hepatitis B vaccine to recommending screening all pregnant individuals for hepatitis B and having a conversation with each pregnant person regarding the risks and benefits of hepatitis B vaccination if the person tests negative (i.e., individual decision-making). If the mother tests positive or their status is unknown, hepatitis B vaccination and a dose of hepatitis B immune globulin would be given to the infant within 12 hours of birth. Critics of this decision cite the safety and efficacy of the hepatitis B vaccine in infants and the 99% drop in annual infections since the implementation of the universal birth dose strategy in 1991.[3] Furthermore, the federal administration has begun implementing changes to align the US childhood vaccination schedule more closely with European models, particularly Denmark's, removing several routine vaccines that had been widely recommended in the United States for decades (https://bit.ly/45duCFR; https://bit.ly/4qpelpT).

The Trump administration has also widely disseminated vaccine information that has been disproven by numerous scientific studies and discredited by highly regarded medical associations. In November 2025, the Centers for Disease Control and Prevention website was altered to question the well-established fact that vaccines do not cause autism, which is supported by more than 40 scientifically sound, large-scale studies.[4] The website also states that the US Department of Health and Human Services has

AJPH March 2026, Vol. 116, No. 3

launched a comprehensive assessment of the causes of autism that will explore the potential association between childhood vaccination and autism. No additional information regarding this proposed assessment is available as of this writing.

The undermining of research that has definitively disproven the link between vaccines and autism has sown doubt and needless confusion among well-intentioned parents who are rightfully concerned about autism and has left many with questions regarding the safety of childhood vaccines. Parental vaccine hesitancy will most likely contribute to decreased uptake of safe and effective childhood vaccines, which was already declining in recent years.[5] Moreover, the US secretary of Health and Human Services has repeatedly stated that parents and caregivers should "do their own research" and therefore carry the undue burden of understanding and digesting complex information before deciding to vaccinate their children.[6]

These events have been met with outrage by the public health community and applause by antivaccine groups. As the nation's premier public health journal, *AJPH* has as its mission to advance evidence-based public health research, policy, practice, and education. We believe reinvestigating a causal link between vaccines and autism given the strength of evidence refuting any association is futile and diverts resources away from other critical priorities. Instead, we support the system of establishing vaccine recommendations that has successfully worked for decades to provide sound vaccine guidance in this country.

Because of the ongoing, rapidly evolving public health challenges, *AJPH* strives to promote discussions of strategies to strengthen and even reimagine public health systems to advance population health, promote health equity, and ensure scientifically sound vaccination recommendations. Our goal is to provide a forum to discuss and document high-quality, accurate science, irrespective of politics or partisanship. For example, the 2026 *AJPH* State of the Public Health Union event demonstrated our commitment to advancing public health by fostering discussions and amplifying diverse voices and opinions across the political spectrum. We explored the current state and possible future directions of the federal public health system, including the development of vaccine recommendations, with distinguished former health leaders from Democratic and Republican federal administrations.

In forthcoming issues, *AJPH* will be publishing a series of invited editorials written by public health leaders and experts representing major national organizations. These editorials will tackle the current challenges the country faces as its governmental public health system undergoes transformation. Authors were invited to discuss what key stakeholders can do to address vaccine access given the recent federal developments. Many editorials will focus on vaccines and vaccination policies, and some will highlight challenges to state and local municipalities as they face funding loss and attempt to maintain necessary public health services.

The first editorial in this series (Higgins; p. 292) provides an overview of the American Academy of Pediatrics' efforts to provide consistent evidence-based guidance in lieu of the recent controversial ACIP recommendations. Future editorials will detail efforts under way by regional state and local collaborations to fill gaps left by reduced funding and support from the federal health agencies. In addition, forthcoming editorials will provide an overview of the health insurance industry's role in increasing access to recommended vaccines.

We have also invited an author to describe the role of US states in protecting public health resources and another to highlight city and county efforts to address vaccine misinformation, advance health equity, and reach undervaccinated local communities. In the future, we may commission articles that provide an overview of European vaccine schedules, shed light on proposed changes to the Food and Drug Administration's vaccine approval process, and address other pressing topics.

We thank the authors of these editorials for their contributions. Our intention is to spur thoughtful, scientifically sound ideas, rigorous research, and evidence-informed actions to protect public health. We are open to accepting and publishing unsolicited editorials that are balanced, that examine one's own position, and that are scientifically accurate to promote ongoing discussions as we work toward solutions that control vaccine preventable diseases and support health and wellness nationally. AJPH

CORRESPONDENCE

Correspondence should be sent to Denys T. Lau, Editor-in-Chief, American Public Health Association, 800 I St NW, Washington, DC 20001 (e-mail: Denys.Lau@apha.org). Reprints can be ordered at https://www.ajph.org by clicking the "Reprints" link.

PUBLICATION INFORMATION

Full Citation: Ojikutu BO, Lau DT. Public health controversies: *AJPH*'s series on public health transformation and vaccines. *Am J Public Health*. 2026;116(3):289–291.

Acceptance Date: January 5, 2026.

DOI: https://doi.org/10.2105/AJPH.2025.308396

CONTRIBUTORS

B. O. Ojikutu drafted and D. T. Lau revised the editorial.

ACKNOWLEDGMENTS

This article is part of an *AJPH* series on vaccine access and vaccination policies. Written by public health experts representing major organizations, these editorials tackle the current challenges the country faces in accessing vaccine care as governmental public health system undergoes transformation. Our intention is to spur thoughtful, scientifically sound ideas, rigorous research, and evidence-informed actions to protect population health. We welcome unsolicited editorials that are balanced, scientifically accurate, and self-reflective in examining one's own position to promote ongoing discussions as we work toward solutions that control vaccine preventable diseases and support health and wellness nationally.

CONFLICTS OF INTEREST

The authors have no conflicts of interest to disclose.

REFERENCES

1. Smith JC, Snider DE, Pickering LK; Advisory Committee on Immunization Practices. Immunization policy development in the United States: the role of the Advisory Committee on Immunization Practices. *Ann Intern Med.* 2009;150(1):45–49. https://doi.org/10.7326/0003-4819-150-1-200901060-00009
2. US Department of Health and Human Services. HHS takes bold step to restore public trust in vaccines by reconstituting ACIP. June 9, 2025. Available at: https://www.hhs.gov/press-room/hhs-restore-public-trust-vaccines-acip.html. Accessed December 20, 2025.
3. Kaiser Family Foundation. Recent changes in federal vaccine recommendations: what's the impact on insurance coverage? December 16, 2025. Available at: https://www.kff.org/other-health/recent-changes-in-federal-vaccine-recommendations-whats-the-impact-on-insurance-coverage. Accessed December 20, 2025.
4. Centers for Disease Control and Prevention. Autism and vaccines. Available at: https://www.cdc.gov/vaccine-safety/about/autism.html. November 19, 2025. Accessed December 20, 2025.
5. Centers for Disease Control and Prevention. Vaccination coverage and exemptions among kindergartners. July 31, 2025. Available at: https://www.cdc.gov/schoolvaxview/data/index.html#cdc_data_surveillance_section_2-new-findings-on-vaccination-coverage-and-exemptions-among-kindergartners-2024-2025-school-year. Accessed January 4, 2026.
6. New York Times. Kennedy advises new parents to "do your own research" on vaccines. Available at: https://www.nytimes.com/2025/04/29/us/politics/kennedy-vaccines-research.html. Accessed January 4, 2026.

Filling the Federal Void Through Shared Leadership in Vaccine Policy

David M. Higgins, MD, MPH

ABOUT THE AUTHOR

David M. Higgins is with the Department of Pediatrics at the University of Colorado School of Medicine, Aurora. He serves as vice president and immunization representative for the Colorado chapter of the American Academy of Pediatrics.

See also Ojikutu and Lau, p. 289.

AJPH March 2026, Vol. 116, No. 3

For over a century, federal public health institutions have played a pivotal role in shaping health policymaking, providing the scientific foundation and unified standards that inform state laws, clinical practice, and equitable access to care. In 2025, a series of federal actions hollowed out that framework, leaving a rapidly growing void at the center of our national health policy.

Nowhere is that impact more visible than in immunization. For six decades, the Centers for Disease Control and Prevention (CDC), guided by the Advisory Committee on Immunization Practices (ACIP), defined the scientific consensus on vaccine safety, effectiveness, and use.[1] Since its first meeting in 1964, the ACIP has provided evidence-based guidance from independent experts on the use of vaccines. Its recommendations have shaped the national immunization schedule, informed insurance coverage and vaccine availability for low-income children, influenced state laws, and bolstered public confidence. Over the past 12 presidential administrations, the ACIP has established itself as the global gold standard for transparent, science-driven vaccine guidance, relied upon by clinicians and regulators worldwide.

That foundation is now being dismantled. In 2025, a new health administration decimated the infrastructure upon which this success was built. Top CDC leaders have either left or been removed from their positions, and the entire ACIP membership has been dismissed and replaced with individuals lacking relevant expertise who did not undergo the standard, rigorous vetting process.[1] The damage extends beyond leadership as critical CDC programs have faced deep funding cuts, degrading the surveillance, analytic, and safety-monitoring capacities that guide national vaccine policy.[2] This erosion of scientific rigor also extends beyond the CDC; the Food and Drug Administration has bypassed key safeguards by issuing new, restrictive labels for COVID-19 vaccines without a transparent, independent review.[3] At the same time, some officials have distorted the idea of "gold-standard science" to justify renewed skepticism of well-established vaccine safety, a message that undermines both evidence and public trust.[4]

As pediatricians, we see the immediate consequences of this uncertainty every day. Parents are asking more than ever whether vaccines are still recommended, covered, or even safe. Providers face confusion about how to advise families amid conflicting guidance. And although most parents want their children to be vaccinated, they are increasingly uncertain as to how and when to do so. The result is gaps in vaccination that leave more children unprotected, increasing the likelihood that diseases rarely seen today, such as measles, invasive *Haemophilus influenzae* type b disease, and pneumococcal meningitis, will return to our clinics and communities.

Against this backdrop, the question is no longer whether the public health community should fill the federal leadership void, but how. That work has already begun. Across the country, a growing constellation of partners has stepped forward to build a new model of distributed public health governance in which policymaking, implementation, and communication are shared responsibilities.

Professional associations have become stabilizers in this fragile moment. Organizations such as the American Academy of Pediatrics (AAP) have long been a scientific authority and trusted voice on topics like immunization, providing expert guidance to complement and reinforce federal recommendations. However, this year their role has shifted fundamentally from supporting federal vaccine guidance to filling the gap left by its absence. When federal recommendations for the current respiratory season were delayed and inconsistent, the AAP issued its own independent, evidence-based immunization schedule.[5] Other professional societies, including the American Academy of Family Physicians, the American College of Obstetricians and

Gynecologists, and the Infectious Diseases Society of America, have taken similar steps, signaling a reorientation of scientific leadership beyond the federal level.[6]

These professional societies and a broad network of immunization partners, including public health agencies, nursing and pharmacy organizations, immunization managers, and nonprofit coalitions, now face three immediate challenges: policy fragmentation, compromised access, and erosion of public trust.

First, states have been compelled to decouple their vaccine-related laws, regulations, and policies from federal guidance to maintain science-based recommendations and continuity of care. Born out of necessity, these swift defensive actions have created a national patchwork of policy that risks deepening existing inequities: childhood vaccine coverage is already lower in rural and low-income families, is lower among children of foreign-born parents compared with those of US-born parents, and varies substantially by race and ethnicity.[7,8] Still, the greater danger lies in inaction; even an inequitable patchwork of state policies is less harmful than allowing preventable harm to occur.

Second, the growing network of partners will need to work together to mitigate compromised vaccine access. For the millions of children who rely on the federally administered Vaccines for Children—the backbone of vaccine equity for low-income and uninsured families that covers roughly half of the children in the United States—any federal ambiguity can disrupt or delay vaccine access and place new financial and logistical burdens on families least able to bear them.

Finally, when vaccine decisions appear to be driven by politics rather than science, already fragile public trust will suffer even more. As federal public messaging becomes increasingly confusing and inconsistent, people turn to social media or online communities for answers—sources that often mix fact with speculation. These challenges highlight the vulnerability of our public health systems, but rebuilding trust and infrastructure from the ground up is already underway.

This unprecedented moment presents an opportunity to build a more resilient, community-centered public health framework for the future. In addition to vaccine policy, partners across the health, public health, and community sectors will need to increasingly assume other roles once supported by federal agencies, including coordinating public communication; strengthening the skills of the public health workforce through shared training, guidance, and technical assistance; and helping states and jurisdictions to align evidence-based public health practices to reduce fragmentation. Some are already building rapid-response communication networks, offering cross-state technical assistance, and developing shared standards.

State and regional coalitions are already assuming roles once supported by federal infrastructure. Regional partnerships such as the West Coast Health Alliance, the Northeast Public Health Collaborative, and the Governors' Public Health Alliance,[6] initiatives such as the Vaccine Integrity Project,[9] as well as numerous state and local efforts like Colorado Chooses Vaccines,[10] show how coordinated local leadership can share knowledge, resources, and expertise across state lines and communities. Their continued collaboration is necessary to sustain public health in the absence of unified federal direction.

Yet, temporizing efforts to fill gaps should not be mistaken for a permanent replacement of federal leadership. No state coalition or professional organization can fully replace the federal systems that approve new vaccines, ensure their safety, finance their research and supply chains, and maintain consistent national standards for coverage and liability. If fixes begin to look permanent, we risk cementing inequities and weakening the federal foundation of our nation's public health.

To meet this moment, the broad public health community, including professional societies, state and regional coalitions, health systems, nonprofit organizations, and local public health agencies, must continue collaborating to protect the continuity of science and the integrity of childhood vaccine health policy. Many of these groups, including the AAP, are already working together to coordinate communication, share evidence, and support clinicians and communities. These actions must include the following three essential priorities.

1. Ensure vaccine access. The public health community must safeguard consistent access to vaccines for children and adults, regardless of shifting federal guidance, while continuing to press for stable federal investment in the data systems, workforce, and financing that sustain vaccine delivery.
2. Mobilize community-level providers and communicators. Equip frontline providers, public health professionals, and other trusted messengers with the resources, training, and messaging support they need to efficiently and effectively counter misinformation and navigate new systems of vaccine and preventive

AJPH March 2026, Vol. 116, No. 3

care delivery, including ready-to-use messaging, decision aids, and evidence summaries for clinicians, community partners, and the public.

3. Center equity. Ensure that next-generation vaccine and health policies close, not widen, gaps in access for low-income, rural, and medically underserved children. The ability to choose vaccination should never depend on a family's zip code or income.

Public health has always been a collective endeavor. As the federal center weakens, those closest to patients and communities are stepping forward to fill the void and reimagining what public health can be. Their work today is not simply a bridge to recovery; it is the foundation for a stronger, more connected, and community-centered public health system of the future. AJPH

CORRESPONDENCE

Correspondence should be sent to David Higgins, MD, MPH, Mail Stop F443, 1890 N. Revere Court, Aurora, CO 80045 (e-mail: David.Higgins@cuanschutz.edu). Reprints can be ordered at https://www.ajph.org by clicking the "Reprints" link.

PUBLICATION INFORMATION

Full Citation: Higgins DM. Filling the federal void through shared leadership in vaccine policy. *Am J Public Health*. 2026;116(3):292–294.

Acceptance Date: November 20, 2025.

DOI: https://doi.org/10.2105/AJPH.2025.308369

ORCID iD:

David M. Higgins https://orcid.org/0000-0003-2130-7442

ACKNOWLEDGMENTS

This article is part of an *AJPH* series on vaccine access and vaccination policies. Written by public health experts representing major organizations, these editorials tackle the current challenges the country faces in accessing vaccine care as governmental public health system undergoes transformation. Our intention is to spur thoughtful, scientifically sound ideas, rigorous research, and evidence-informed actions to protect population health. We welcome unsolicited editorials that are balanced, scientifically accurate, and self-reflective in examining one's own position to promote ongoing discussions as we work toward solutions that control vaccine preventable diseases and support health and wellness nationally.

See Ojikutu and Lau, available at: https://ajph.aphapublications.org/doi/epub/10.2105/AJPH.2026.308396.

CONFLICTS OF INTEREST

The author has no conflicts of interest to disclose.

REFERENCES

1. Asturias EJ, Brewer NT, Brooks O, et al. Advisory Committee on Immunization Practices at a crossroads. *JAMA*. 2025;334(8):667–668. https://doi.org/10.1001/jama.2025.10776
2. Gostin LO, Lurie P. Assault on the Centers for Disease Control and Prevention—budget cuts, political control, and the erosion of trust. *JAMA Health Forum*. 2025;6(10):e255467. https://doi.org/10.1001/jamahealthforum.2025.5467
3. Vaccine Integrity Project staff and advisers. Viewpoint: making key COVID vaccine decisions without input, transparency is a public disservice. Vaccine Integrity Project, Center for Infectious Disease Research & Policy, University of Minnesota. Available at: https://www.cidrap.umn.edu/covid-19/viewpoint-making-key-covid-vaccine-decisions-without-input-transparency-public-disservice. Accessed November 12, 2025.
4. Caplan A, Pasadyn FL, Mamo N. Fool's-gold science: the ethical and scientific perils of testing most vaccines using placebo-controlled randomized trials. *EMBO Rep*. 2025;26(16):3979–3981. https://doi.org/10.1038/s44319-025-00530-5
5. American Academy of Pediatrics. AAP immunization schedule. Available at: https://publications.aap.org/redbook/resources/15585?autologincheck=redirected#xd_co_f=YTQwMGJjNjgtNTRkMS00NzhiLThjYzgtY2E5ZmJjZTYwMmY4~. Accessed November 12, 2025.
6. National Foundation for Infectious Diseases. Staying on track: evidence-based vaccine recommendations. Available at: https://www.nfid.org/staying-on-track-evidence-based-vaccine-recommendations. Accessed November 12, 2025.
7. Hill HA, Chen M, Elam-Evans LD, Yankey D, Singleton JA. Vaccination coverage by age 24 months among children born during 2018–2019—National Immunization Survey-Child, United States, 2019–2021. *MMWR Morb Mortal Wkly Rep*. 2023;72(2):33–38. https://doi.org/10.15585/mmwr.mm7202a3
8. Tasslimi A, Bell TR, Moore TP, DeBolt C, Ibrahim A, Matheson J. Vaccine coverage at 36 months and 7 years by parental birth country, Washington State. *Pediatrics*. 2024;153(6):e2023064626. https://doi.org/10.1542/peds.2023-064626
9. Center for Infectious Disease Research and Policy. Vaccine Integrity Project—providing trusted, science-based information to empower individuals, families, communities, clinicians, and policymakers to make informed vaccine choices. University of Minnesota. Available at: https://www.cidrap.umn.edu/vaccine-integrity-project?utm_source=chatgpt.com. Accessed November 12, 2025.
10. Rose Community Foundation. Colorado chooses vaccines coalition created in response to federal disruptions. Available at: https://rcfdenver.org/insights/news-article/colorado-chooses-vaccines-coalition-created-in-response-to-federal-disruptions. Accessed November 12, 2025.

October 2025 Attempted Workforce Reduction Puts US Principal Health Statistics Agency at Risk

Jennifer D. Schoendorf, PhD, and Denys T. Lau, PhD

ABOUT THE AUTHORS

Jennifer Schoendorf is AJPH *senior deputy editor and is with the School of Public Health, University of Maryland, College Park. Denys T. Lau is the editor-in-chief of* AJPH *and is with Johns Hopkins University, Bloomberg School of Public Health, Baltimore, MD, the Milken Institute of Public Health, George Washington University, Washington, DC, and the Retzky College of Pharmacy, University of Illinois, Chicago.*

On October 10, 2025, about 4200 federal workers in at least seven agencies unexpectedly received reduction in force (RIF) notices during the US federal government shutdown.[1] The October RIFs followed two previous rounds in which substantial amounts of funding and numbers of personnel were reduced—or, worse, eliminated—affecting federal data systems. Some of these earlier cuts were made to the Substance Abuse and Mental Health Services Administration's National Survey on Substance Use, the Centers for Disease Control and Prevention's Pregnancy Risk Monitoring System, the US Department of Agriculture's monitoring of food insecurity, and nearly the entire National Center for Education Statistics.

In the latest round of RIFs, federal workers who were laid off included more than 100 employees from the nation's principal health statistics agency—the National Center for Health Statistics (NCHS) at the Centers for Disease Control and Prevention (nearly 25% of its workforce). By mid-November, as a condition of a congressionally negotiated spending bill to reopen the federal government, many of the October layoff notices were rescinded. However, the public health community witnessed how fragile our nation's federal statistics ecosystem is and how easily essential information needed for policy and decision-making could become compromised.

As former federal workers, we—the authors of this editorial—spent our careers measuring and tracking the health of the US population and knew that the data collected and statistics provided by federal statistics agencies enabled policymakers to make informed decisions with objective information in hand. We were proud to see our work featured in various policy reports, news articles, and research articles and to hear it referenced by decision-makers and policy leaders. In this editorial, we focus on NCHS, the agency we know the best.

Although NCHS is a relatively small agency, the statistical information that it produces touches everyday lives. News coverage frequently reports on overdose deaths in the United States, declining birth rates, and obesity trends. These and many other national health statistics are collected, compiled, and published by NCHS. Trends in the number of people with chronic conditions often come from NCHS' National Health Interview Survey. The current administration frequently cites statistics about consumption of ultraprocessed foods and exposure to environmental toxins from NCHS' National Health and Nutrition Examination Survey.[2] Statistics about services used in emergency departments, hospitals, and other health care settings often come from NCHS' family of national health care surveys. Many articles in *AJPH* and other scholarly journals cite official statistics from NCHS to provide motivation and context for their research questions. Another large body of scientific research uses NCHS data to directly answer public health questions.

Like so many, we cannot explain the motivation behind the recent efforts in funding and workforce reductions aimed at NCHS and other federal data programs. After all, the administration fully used NCHS data in their Make America Healthy Again reports on life expectancy, chronic conditions, suicide, chemical exposures, and allergies.[2] The authors of the Make America Healthy Again reports might not have recognized that NCHS provided many of the US statistics cited in the reports' key references from the Organization for Economic Cooperation and Development, the World Health Organization, the Commonwealth Fund, and other sources.

The authors' oversight may be attributable to the wide variety of data available everywhere. If you ask ChatGPT how many people in the United States have diabetes, it will give you an answer that would likely be the latest reported number from NCHS. Without NCHS,

AJPH March 2026, Vol. 116, No. 3

ChatGPT would provide an answer based on other sources: published research studies, online polls and posts, and reports from various governmental, private, and media organizations. However, these other sources are not intended to provide national health estimates. Although federal statistics programs are required to provide guidance about the quality and utility of their data, other sources may not fully document methods, statistical biases, and undue influences. Oftentimes, privately owned data can be proprietary, reducing generalizability, replicability, and transparency.

At first glance, the October RIFs at NCHS may not appear to have had a significant impact because most of the data program staff working directly with the health data were left intact. An exception was the National Death Index staff, who standardize and link national mortality data to other key data for scientific studies and evaluation.[3,4] However, a closer look would reveal that a large number of the behind-the-scenes staff who support the data programs were targeted to be laid off, including those who uphold the legal data security and infrastructure standards, the statistical and methodological research staff who ensure the scientific integrity of the data, and the communication staff who ensure that released information is clearly presented and free of political bias.

Things may have changed after January 31, 2026, when the temporary suspension on RIF actions was scheduled to be lifted. However, the October RIFs have shaken the public health community by reminding us that our public health data and the supporting infrastructure are highly susceptible to political shifts. The trustworthiness of public health data could be called into question if political ideology is not kept out of the collection and dissemination of our nation's official statistics.[5]

In addition to funding cuts to hinder future data collections and RIF actions to limit or terminate support for federal health data programs, the administration had attempted to erase archived data by removing years of data, selected survey variables, and survey documentations from many government Web sites.[6] These attempts were thwarted by recent lawsuits (e.g., by AcademyHealth and the City of San Francisco) to reinstate removed federal data from Web pages.[7,8] Nonetheless, limiting statistical information about sensitive topics, such as gender identify, means that policy decisions cannot be informed or be held accountable using objective data. Furthermore, the erasure and termination of data resources reduce the ability of public health scientists to answer key research questions aimed at moving our knowledge forward.

The COVID-19 pandemic uncovered weaknesses in our public health data infrastructure and strained its capacity. However, that crisis also galvanized discussions on developing and implementing innovations.[9] Optimistically, there is an opportunity to recommit ourselves to robust programs for national health data to guide decisions and evaluate their impact. Public and private leaders are coming together to try to preserve, protect, and innovate public health data ecosystems at state and local levels.[10,11] These preservation and innovation strategies are aimed at ensuring that public health leaders continue making important decisions using accurate, up-to-date, objective information.

Professionals in all trades know the value of the right tools for their craft. Just as chefs are more likely to use high-quality knives to get their dishes just right, decision-makers who rely on national health data need unbiased, accurate, and relevant data to make the best decisions. Although we can disagree and debate the relative importance of obesity and chemical exposures for the health of the US population or the best way to deliver health care equitably across the country, these important policy decisions should not be blurred by confusion on how many of us are overweight, how many of us have detectable levels of lead in our bodies, or how many of us do not have health insurance—counts that are made available through NCHS data. As the former US senator Daniel Patrick Moynihan (D, NY) said, "Everyone is entitled to [their] own opinion, but not [their] own facts." AJPH

CORRESPONDENCE

Correspondence should be sent to Denys T. Lau, Editor-in-Chief, American Public Health Association, 800 I St NW, Washington, DC 20001 (e-mail: Denys.Lau@apha.org). Reprints can be ordered at https://www.ajph.org by clicking the "Reprints" link.

PUBLICATION INFORMATION

Full Citation: Schoendorf JD, Lau DT. October 2025 attempted workforce reduction puts US principal health statistics agency at risk. *Am J Public Health*. 2026;116(3):295–297.

Acceptance Date: January 7, 2026.

DOI: https://doi.org/10.2105/AJPH.2025.308403

CONTRIBUTORS

J. D. Schoendorf drafted and D. T. Lau revised the editorial.

CONFLICTS OF INTEREST

The authors have no conflicts of interest to disclose.

REFERENCES

1. Fowler S, Hsu A, Simmons-Duffin S, Gringlas S, Shivaram D. Trump administration says about 4,200 federal employees face layoffs. October 10, 2025. Available at: https://www.npr.org/2025/10/10/nx-s1-5570933/shutdown-federal-workers-rifs-layoffs-vought#:~:text=More%20than%20a%20week%20into,the%20Democrats%2C%22%20Trump%20said. Accessed January 12, 2026.

2. White House. MAHA report. Available at: https://www.whitehouse.gov/wp-content/uploads/2025/05/MAHA-Report-The-White-House.pdf. Accessed January 12, 2026.
3. Schoendorf JD, Rothwell C. Letter to the editor. *Washington Post.* November 10, 2025. Available at: https://www.washingtonpost.com/opinions/2025/11/10/veterans-affairs-ndi-puerto-rico. Accessed January 12, 2026.
4. Centers for Disease Control and Prevention. National Death Index. July 18, 2024. Available at: https://www.cdc.gov/nchs/ndi/index.html. Accessed January 1, 2026.
5. Bendavid N. Government's historic role as trusted information source is under threat. December 20, 2025. *Washington Post.* Available at: https://www.washingtonpost.com/politics/2025/12/20/data-information-federal-government-trump. Accessed January 12, 2026.
6. Steenhuysen J, Hesson T. US health agencies scrub HIV, other data to remove "gender ideology." January 31, 2025. Available at: https://www.reuters.com/world/us/us-health-agencies-scrub-hiv-other-data-remove-gender-ideology-2025-02-01. Accessed January 12, 2026.
7. City Attorney of San Francisco. Federal government restores access to critical public health data after SF wins lawsuit. December 22, 2025. Available at: https://sfcityattorney.org/federal-government-restores-access-to-critical-public-health-data-after-sf-wins-lawsuit. Accessed January 12, 2026.
8. AcademyHealth. AcademyHealth data lawsuit settlement: key facts and outcomes. Available at: https://academyhealth.org/sites/default/files/publication/%5Bfield_date%3Acustom%3AY%5D-%5Bfield_date%3Acustom%3Am%5D/ah_lawsuit_key_facts.pdf. Accessed January 12, 2026.
9. Lau DT, Sosa P, Dasgupta N, He H. Impact of the COVID-19 pandemic on public health surveillance and survey data collections in the United States. *Am J Public Health.* 2021;111(12):2118–2121. https://doi.org/10.2105/AJPH.2021.306551
10. Varma JK. How states and cities can defend public health in 2026. December 11, 2025. Available at: https://www.healthbeat.org/2025/12/11/local-public-health-supplies-stockpiles-laws. Accessed January 12, 2026.
11. Dasgupta N, Schoendorf JD, Lau DT, Thorpe L. Public trust, private data: four considerations for the future of health. *Am J Public Health.* 2026;116(1):57–61. https://doi.org/10.2105/AJPH.2025.308328

AJPH
A PUBLICATION OF THE AMERICAN PUBLIC HEALTH ASSOCIATION

Call for Papers

AJPH SPECIAL SECTION ON BEREAVEMENT AS A GLOBAL HEALTH CONCERN

AJPH has issued a Call for Papers to seek original research, analytic essays, history essays, notes from the field, and opinion editorials that address the central question:

Considering current global events, how does bereavement function differently across subgroups, either as a cause or a consequence of population health outcomes?

Submissions are due on March 1, 2026.

Although socio-political factors may frame the experience of death and bereavement, we are interested in scientific papers that are primarily focused on bereavement within diverse global contexts and populations. We seek papers that address, but are not limited to, the following topics:

- Population distribution of bereavement and how it is changing over time.
- Impacts of specific sources or contexts of bereavement.
- Exposure to bereavement in the workplace.
- Factors on resilience to bereavement effects.
- Experiences across cultures and influence on health outcomes.
- Effects on mental and physical health.
- Improved measures to reflect cross-cultural experiences.
- Interventions that successfully minimize health impacts.
- Policies/practices to serve diverse needs of bereaved populations.
- Bereavement service gaps across the globe.
- Scientific evidence on best practices in providing bereavement services.

AJPH seeks original research articles, notes from the field, analytic essays, and opinion editorials that are data-driven, timely, unbiased, and thorough in their methods and interpretation, as well as opinion editorials that are well-balanced, self-reflective (i.e., examines one's own position), and scientifically accurate. **Read the full call for papers at https://ajph.aphapublications.org/callforpapers.**

Potential authors should visit the *AJPH* website (www.ajph.org) to review the Instructions for Authors. Importantly, submissions must include a cover letter formatted as requested and should specify that the submission is for the "Bereavement as a Public Health Concern" special section. In all manuscripts, the number of words, references, and tables/figures must correspond to a specific *AJPH* article format. **Submissions are due on March 1, 2026**, and can be submitted at https://www.editorialmanager.com/ajph. If you have any questions, please contact Dr. Michelle Livings, *AJPH* Assistant Editor, at **michelle.livings@rutgers.edu.**

***AJPH* Editors**: *Michelle Livings and Emily Smith-Greenaway*

Transgender and Gender-Diverse Rights and Health: A Global Perspective

Mauro Cabral Grinspan, Lic, and Sofia Gruskin, JD, MIA

ABOUT THE AUTHORS

Mauro Cabral Grinspan was with the Free University of Brussels at the time of this editorial. Sofia Gruskin is with the Institute on Inequalities in Global Health, Keck School of Medicine and Gould School of Law, University of Southern California.

AJPH March 2026, Vol. 116, No. 3

In their article "Contextualizing President Trump's Executive Orders Targeting Transgender Health and Gender-Affirming Care: How Did We Get Here?," Nuruzzaman and Hsiang provide a nuanced account of the current state of emergency in the field of transgender medicine in the United States and the growing challenges transgender and gender-diverse people in the country are confronting in accessing both general and gender-affirming health care.[1] While acknowledging the specificity of the US situation, we believe the scale of those challenges, and the accompanying antigender rhetoric, are most usefully addressed not in isolation but as part of a broader international campaign against sexual diversity, gender equality, and human rights.

Transgender and gender-diverse people and their access to health care are under attack from far-right influencers, including certain media outlets and some feminist and lesbian, gay, and bisexual organizations,[2] as well as some religious institutions, "concerned parents," and sitting governments[3] in all regions of the world.[4] Focused on protecting the world against so-called "gender ideology," those actors work against comprehensive sexuality education, contraception and abortion, same-sex marriage and adoption, surrogacy, sex work, and the very existence of transgender and gender-diverse people.[5] This antitrans rhetoric is intrinsically linked to other regressive agendas tied to migration, racial justice, and the climate crisis, forming a shared politics of reaction against perceived threats to outdated traditional hierarchies and social control.

The global movement against transgender and gender-diverse people is having a negative impact even in those countries that had positive legal and regulatory changes in recent years. Argentina's 2012 Gender Identity Law[6] set a global precedent for national-level recognition of self-determination and access to gender-affirming health care allowing individuals to change legal gender markers without medical or juridical gatekeeping, while guaranteeing access to gender-affirming health care through the public health system based on informed consent. Many other countries and jurisdictions followed this example. Since the beginning of his presidency, however, Javier Milei has sought to pass a restrictive amendment to the law or to derogate from it entirely. Countries that used to require sterilization to grant access to legal gender recognition, such as The Netherlands[7] and Sweden,[8] have in recent years publicly apologized for these human rights violations and established compensation programs for affected individuals. Both countries are now ruled by right-wing governments, and the health and human rights of transgender and gender-diverse people living there are once again at risk.

At the global level, the World Health Organization (WHO) adoption of the *International Classification of Diseases, 11th Revision* (*ICD-11*) in 2019 represented a significant milestone in depathologization. The *ICD-11,* on the basis of evidence and medical consensus, removed transgender-related categories for adults from the chapter on mental and behavioral disorders, reclassifying "gender identity disorder" as "gender incongruence" within a new chapter on sexual health.[9] Not surprisingly, both WHO and its work on transgender and gender-diverse issues have been under relentless attack by antigender actors in recent years. The same can be said of assaults against the World Professional Association for Transgender Health, all in a broader context where scientific evidence is increasingly degraded to a matter of opinion.

With respect to international human rights standards, there have been growing protections to support the rights of transgender and gender-diverse people at global level. Perhaps most importantly, the Yogyakarta Principles (2006) and Yogyakarta Principles Plus 10 (2017) articulate how existing international human rights law applies to sexual orientation, gender identity, gender expression, and sex characteristics.[10] These documents do not create new rights or create new obligations but clarify how *already existing* human rights standards can be applied to sexual orientation, gender identity, gender expression, and sex characteristics. Strategic use of these international standards has supported domestic legal reforms and judicial decisions in multiple jurisdictions. Current opposition to these developments can be understood as part of the larger backlash seeking to weaken the legitimacy of global human rights institutions and the multilateral system more broadly.

Transgender and gender-diverse people around the world are now facing a threefold health crisis: First, their access to gender-affirming treatments is being severely restricted or denied, and in some jurisdictions even criminalized. Second, their access to general health care is increasingly threatened, compounded not only by the transphobia that exists in many health care settings but also by the ways this intersects with poverty, racism, xenophobia, and other forms of discrimination. Third, their very physical and mental health and well-being is often under attack, impaired by the stigma, discrimination and violence happening against them and their communities.[11]

Understanding how we arrived at this crisis requires recognizing its global scope and ideological coherence. Yet, as important as the question of how we got here is the question of how we get out of here. Current circumstances demand the internationalization of these efforts—for example, by integrating international human rights standards and supporting health care system reform toward universal health coverage. Activists worldwide are developing emancipatory strategies grounded in collective mobilization, collaborative initiatives,[12] and transnational solidarity.[13]

Confronting what is happening to transgender and gender-diverse people in the United States requires addressing the global dimension of the processes at stake, engaging with the movements advancing global responses to those processes, and recognizing that national reforms alone will never be sufficient to secure lasting protection. Building inclusive health systems, reaffirming international human rights standards, and joining collective political efforts beyond national borders are essential steps to ensure dignity, equality, and justice for all. AJPH

CORRESPONDENCE

Correspondence should be sent to Mauro Cabral Grinspan, STRIGES, Maison des Sciences Humaines, Campus Solbosch, Free University of Brussels Rue Arthur Diderich 69, Bruxelles, 1060, BELGIUM (e-mail: mcabralgrinspan@gmail.com). Reprints can be ordered at https://www.ajph.org by clicking the "Reprints" link.

PUBLICATION INFORMATION

Full Citation: Grinspan MC, Gruskin S. Transgender and gender-diverse rights and health: a global perspective. *Am J Public Health*. 2026;116(3): 298–299.

Acceptance Date: December 16, 2025.

DOI: https://doi.org/10.2105/AJPH.2025.308391

ORCID iDs:

Mauro Cabral Grinspan https://orcid.org/0009-0005-5643-1904

Sofia Gruskin https://orcid.org/0000-0002-2418-011X

CONTRIBUTORS

Both authors contributed equally to the work.

CONFLICTS OF INTEREST

The authors declare no conflict of interest.

REFERENCES

1. Nuruzzaman N, Hsiang E. Contextualizing President Trump's executive orders targeting transgender health and gender-affirming care. *Am J Public Health*. 2026;116(2):256–260. https://doi.org/10.2105/AJPH.2025.308265
2. Vincent B, Erikainen S, Pearce R. *TERF Wars: Feminism and the Fight for Transgender Futures*. London, England: SAGE; 2020.
3. Trump D. Defending Women From Gender Ideology Extremism and Restoring Biological Truth to the Federal Government. The White House. January 20, 2025. Available at: https://www.whitehouse.gov/presidential-actions/2025/01/defending-women-from-gender-ideology-extremism-and-restoring-biological-truth-to-the-federal-government. Accessed December 2, 2025.
4. Global Action for Trans Equality. *The Impact of Anti-Gender Opposition: Global and Regional Reports*. February 21, 2024. Available at: https://gate.ngo/knowledge-portal/news/anti-gender-opposition-impact-global-regional-reports. Accessed December 2, 2025.
5. Paternotte D. Victor Frankenstein and its creature: the many lives of 'gender ideology.' *Int Rev Sociol*. 2023;33(2):80–104. https://doi.org/10.1080/03906701.2023.2187833
6. Argentinean Ministry of Public Finances. Argentina's Gender Identity Law as approved by the Senate of Argentina on May 8, 2012 [English translation]. USC Global Health. Published May 8, 2012. Available at: https://globalhealth.usc.edu/wp-content/uploads/2017/03/english-translation-of-argentina_s-gender-identity-law-as-approved-by-the-senate-of-argentina-on-may-8-2012.pdf. Accessed November 27, 2025.
7. Knight K. Netherlands apologizes for transgender sterilizations. Human Rights Watch. December 1, 2020. Available at: https://www.hrw.org/news/2020/12/01/netherlands-apologizes-transgender-sterilizations. Accessed December 2, 2025.
8. International Lesbian, Gay, Bisexual, Trans and Intersex Association–Europe. Swedish Parliament to pay compensation for forced sterilisation of trans people. March 22, 2018. Available at: https://www.ilga-europe.org/news/wedish-parliament-to-pay-compensation-for-forced-sterilisation-of-trans-people. Accessed November 27, 2025.
9. Cabral Grinspan M, *Eppur si muove*. Reflections on Human Rights and Trans Depathologization in *ICD-11*. In: Chase A, Mahdavi P, Banai H, Gruskin S, eds. *Human Rights at the Intersections. Transformation Through Local, Global and Cosmopolitan Challenges*. London, England: Bloomsbury Academic; 2022.
10. The Yogyakarta Principles on the Application of International Human Rights Law in relation to Sexual Orientation and Gender Identity. March 2007. Available at: https://www.yogyakartaprinciples.org. Accessed November 27, 2025.
11. Rowlands S. *Landscape Analysis: What We Know on Anti-Gender Movement Measures and Actors Targeting Trans People Across Europe and Central Asia*. Trans Europe and Central Asia. Available at: https://tgeu.org/files/uploads/2024/08/TGEU-AGM-landscape-analysis_updated.pdf. Accessed December 2, 2025.
12. An Affirmation of Feminist Principles. Sign-on letter. Available at: https://www.feministaffirmation.org/letter. Accessed November 27, 2025.
13. Trans Justice Project. Statement of solidarity. March 5, 2025. Available at: https://transjustice.org.au/solidarity. Accessed November 27, 2025.

Measure Racism, Not Just Race: Recommendations for Scientific Practice

Felicity T. Enders, PhD, MPH, Philip M. Alberti, PhD, Elizabeth H. Golembiewski, PhD, MPH, Minerva A. Orellana, PhD, MS, Paula Braveman, MD, MPH, Virginia A. Brown, PhD, MA, Nyasha Chambwe, PhD, Chandra L. Ford, PhD, MPH, MLIS, and Joyce E. Balls-Berry, PhD, MPE

ABOUT THE AUTHORS

Felicity T. Enders is a professor of Biostatistics and Clinical and Translational Science at the Mayo Clinic College of Medicine and Science in Rochester, MN. Philip M. Alberti is senior director, health equity research and policy and founding director of the AAMC Center for Health Justice at the Association of American Medical Colleges in Washington, DC. Elizabeth H. Golembiewski is a health services analyst in the Department of Quantitative Health Sciences at Mayo Clinic, Rochester. Minerva A. Orellana is a postdoctoral research fellow in the Department of Obstetrics and Gynecology at the University of Washington in Seattle. Paula Braveman is professor emeritus in the Department of Family and Community Medicine and founding director of the Center for Health Equity at the University of California, San Francisco. Virginia A. Brown is a research scholar at The Hastings Center in Garrison, NY. Nyasha Chambwe is an assistant professor in the Institute for Molecular Medicine at the Feinstein Institutes for Medical Research at Northwell Health in Manhasset, NY. Chandra L. Ford is a professor in the departments of Behavioral, Social and Health Education Sciences and African American Studies at Emory University in Atlanta, GA. Joyce E. Balls-Berry is an associate professor in the Department of Neurology at Washington University School of Medicine in St Louis, MO.

Note. The views and opinions expressed in this article are those of the authors and do not necessarily reflect the views of their institutions or their affiliates.

An urgent need exists for scientific practices that explicitly measure racism, not just race, as a key driver of health disparities. Racism is a systemic force that structures opportunity and assigns value based on perceived racial phenotypes, disadvantaging some, advantaging others, and undermining societal well-being by wasting human potential.[1] Despite overwhelming evidence of its impact, racism is often denied or minimized and remains deeply embedded in US institutions, shaping inequities in health, education, housing, and economic opportunity.[2]

Within the scientific enterprise, racism influences every stage of research: from study design and recruitment to analysis and dissemination. It operates both overtly, through discriminatory funding and exclusionary practices, and covertly, through methodologies and assumptions that appear neutral but reinforce injustice. Building on a growing body of scholarship on the role of "race" in research,[3–6] this editorial provides research-informed, practical recommendations to support a shift in scientific practice: one that rejects flawed uses of race and centers the measurable impacts of racism on health and well-being. By replacing outdated defaults and developing stronger analytic frameworks, science can advance equity, accuracy, and accountability.

WHY RACISM, NOT RACE?

Race is often treated in research as if it were a fixed biological trait, a practice both scientifically inaccurate and ethically harmful. In reality, race is a sociopolitical classification rooted in systems of oppression, not biology. When race is used as a proxy for genetic difference, researchers risk conflating deeply embedded social processes with innate physiological traits, reinforcing racial essentialism, misdirecting analysis, and obscuring the actual drivers of health inequities.

Racism—not race—produces and sustains health disparities.[7] In most cases, "race" as a variable in research reflects unmeasured exposures to racism, like structural factors, discrimination, and socioeconomic disadvantage. Therefore, measuring racism involves capturing its effects through variables related to residential segregation, discriminatory policies, chronic stress exposure, and inequitable access to education, employment, or health care.[8] Here, we use "structural racism" to refer to the policies, institutions, and systems that generate inequity and "systemic racism" to describe how these structures collectively reinforce one another across society.

USES OF "RACE" IN SCIENTIFIC RESEARCH

When race is included as a predictor variable in models without clear justification, as is standard practice, it reinforces biological essentialism and obscures the structural and social mechanisms that drive health disparities.[9,10] As illustrated in Figure 1, the uncritical use of "race" has become embedded in the very DNA of scientific inquiry, replicating structural racism within research and clinical practice.[11]

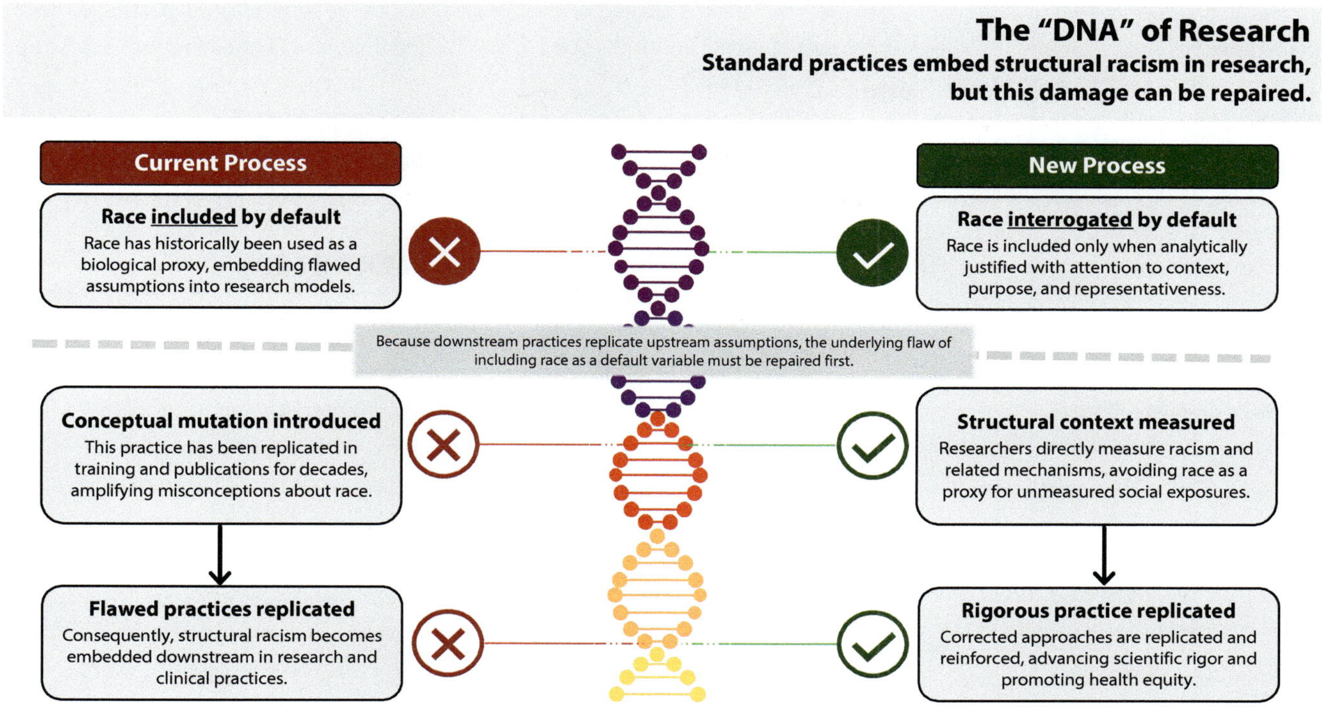

FIGURE 1— A Conceptual Illustration Using DNA as a Metaphor to Contrast Current and Proposed Research Practices Related to Race and Racism

Note. The left panel depicts how the routine inclusion of race as a biological proxy without clear analytic justification functions as a conceptual "mutation," embedding structural racism into scientific inquiry and clinical practice. These flawed practices are perpetuated through ongoing replication across training, publication, and policy. The right panel illustrates a restructured approach: researchers explicitly interrogate the rationale for including race in analytic models and emphasize structural context and racism as measurable exposures.

Conversely, when race is used within race- or racism-conscious study designs, which explicitly examine how racism impacts health through social, structural, and systemic pathways rather than biological difference, it can serve as a valuable entry point for understanding how systems of oppression manifest and operate across health contexts.[6] The continued use of race remains essential for assessing sample representativeness and for examining how the impacts of racism vary across different racialized populations.

RECOMMENDATIONS FOR USING RACE AND MEASURING RACISM

To advance equity-oriented science, researchers must define the purpose of including race and prioritize direct measurement of racism. The following recommendations offer practical guidance:

1. Avoid using race as a predictor variable unless explicitly conducting race- or racism-conscious research. In rare cases where biological differences correlate with racialized categories, use direct biological measures instead of race. If the aim is to assess the impact of racism, include variables that capture racism directly rather than using race as a proxy. Exclude race from machine-learning models by default. Uncritical use of race in predictive models can reinforce bias, especially when data on racialized populations are incomplete or unrepresentative.[12]
2. Use race to assess sample representativeness and generalizability, using at minimum the seven US Office of Management and Budget categories: American Indian or Alaska Native, Asian, Black or African American, Hispanic or Latino, Middle Eastern or North African, Native Hawaiian or Pacific Islander, and White. Disaggregate further where appropriate.
3. Include socioeconomic status or related concepts, but do not treat them as substitutes for racism. Socioeconomic status often mediates or moderates the effects of racism. Treating it solely as a confounder can mask the structural drivers of

inequity. Refer to recent National Academies guidance and the National Institutes of Health PhenX Toolkit for validated measures of these and other concepts.[6]

4. Assess whether adding or stratifying by race improves model performance. If race improves model fit, report both models and interpret differences through a racism-conscious lens. Any remaining disparities are likely due to unmeasured effects of racism, not biological distinctions. In rare cases where biological differences are associated with racialized categories, researchers must take care to avoid reinforcing racial essentialism.

A DEEPER ASSESSMENT OF RACISM: GUIDING QUESTIONS

To study the effects of racism rigorously, researchers must move beyond proxies and engage with the lived, structural, and systemic dimensions of racism. The following guiding questions support deeper inquiry. Emphasizing *here* underscores that racism manifests differently across environments and communities. These questions are intended as a flexible foundation for measure development, research design, and community collaboration, and may be adapted or expanded based on study context.

1. How might racism be operating *here*?
   - What forms of racism may be present in this context?
   - What mechanisms (e.g., intrapersonal, interpersonal, organizational, and societal) enable racism?
   - Which structures, policies, practices, norms, and values drive inequities?
   - Who is affected most by racism?
   - Is racism causing avoidable, unjust inequities in health outcomes, community conditions, or access to vital services?
   - How does racism affect experiences within systems like health care or education?
   - Are opportunities structured differentially by race?
   - Across sectors (e.g., health, education, economics) and domains (e.g., leadership, productivity, creativity), how does racism diminish collective societal strength?
   - Are there efforts to deny or ignore racism?
2. How do we intervene to dismantle racism *here*?
   - What structures, policies, practices, norms, and values could facilitate equitable opportunity?
   - How can intervention points be identified and leveraged?
   - How can communities and stakeholders be meaningfully engaged?
   - What strategies can incorporate diverse perspectives into antiracism efforts?
   - How can this work align with ethical principles and community priorities?

Measuring racism is necessarily more complex than measuring race. Racism operates across interconnected structural, institutional, interpersonal, and internalized pathways, which rarely map neatly onto single variables. To support researchers, we suggest several strategies to capture racism's operation without oversimplification: pairing multilevel data with community expertise, combining policy and environmental indicators with individual experiences, using validated indices where available, and explicitly theorizing mechanisms in causal diagrams.

NEXT STEPS

Eliminating racism from science requires a fundamental shift in research practice and accountability across the research ecosystem. Researchers should align study design, analysis, and dissemination with antiracist practices. Journal editors should adopt standards requiring clarity in how race is used and whether racism is measured. Scientific reviewers and funders should assess whether proposals avoid reinforcing structural bias, though these recommendations arise at a time when federal priorities regarding structural racism research are shifting, including recent actions to pause or revoke awards focused on structural determinants. Educators should train future scientists to recognize and challenge racism in research. Finally, academic institutions should engage communities to ensure that antiracist values are embedded in scientific leadership.

Critically, this work must also attend to other forms of oppression, such as those based on gender, ability, sexual orientation, and socioeconomic status, which intersect with racism and contribute to unjust outcomes. Addressing these forces collectively is essential for creating a just, inclusive scientific enterprise.

As the saying goes, "What gets measured gets managed." But current norms fail to capture the root causes of inequity. Instead, they obscure or reinforce racism's role in shaping health outcomes. By focusing research on structural and systemic drivers of inequity, science can more accurately identify underlying mechanisms of health disparities, develop targeted interventions, and inform policies that ensure all communities have a fair and just opportunity to thrive. AJPH

CORRESPONDENCE

Correspondence should be sent to Felicity T. Enders, PhD, Minnesota BioBusiness Center, Room 575, Rochester, MN 55902 (e-mail: enders.felicity@mayo.edu). Reprints can be ordered at https://www.ajph.org by clicking the "Reprints" link.

PUBLICATION INFORMATION

Full Citation: Enders FT, Alberti PM, Golembiewski EH, et al. Measure racism, not just race: recommendations for scientific practice. *Am J Public Health*. 2026;116(3):300–303.

Acceptance Date: December 15, 2025.

DOI: https://doi.org/10.2105/AJPH.2025.308393

ORCID iDs:

Felicity T. Enders https://orcid.org/0000-0002-3261-5400

Philip M. Alberti https://orcid.org/0000-0002-3381-4882

Elizabeth H. Golembiewski https://orcid.org/0000-0003-1015-3935

Minerva A. Orellana https://orcid.org/0000-0002-0152-7117

Nyasha Chambwe https://orcid.org/0000-0002-2812-0122

Chandra L. Ford https://orcid.org/0000-0001-7684-1840

Joyce E. Balls-Berry https://orcid.org/0000-0003-3497-1115

CONTRIBUTORS

All authors contributed substantially to this work. For concept and design or analysis and interpretation of data, F. T. Enders, P. M. Alberti, and J. E. Balls-Berry organized and moderated the "Measure Racism, Not Just Race" meeting in May 2024; E. H. Golembiewski and M. A. Orellana conducted notetaking and data collection; and F. T. Enders, P. M. Alberti, P. Braveman, V. A. Brown, N. Chambwe, C. L. Ford, and J. E. Balls-Berry led sessions and provided intellectual contributions during the meeting. For drafting or revising the article, F. T. Enders, P. M. Alberti, and E. H. Golembiewski led the initial drafting; M. A. Orellana, P. Braveman, V. A. Brown, N. Chambwe, C. L. Ford, and J. E. Balls-Berry provided substantial feedback; and F. T. Enders and E. H. Golembiewski integrated revisions, prepared the final article, and coordinated submission. All authors approved the final version of the article.

ACKNOWLEDGMENTS

The authors gratefully acknowledge both the Cold Spring Harbor Laboratory's Banbury Center and the participants of the "Measure Racism, Not Just Race" meeting convened at the Banbury Center in May 2024. The insights and discussions from this gathering helped inform the development of the guidelines and recommendations presented in this paper. We especially wish to recognize the contributions of David A. Ansell, MD, MPH, Camara P. Jones, MD, PhD, MPH, Amy J. H. Kind, MD, PhD, Ilan H. Meyer, PhD, and Somava Saha, MD, MS.

CONFLICTS OF INTEREST

The authors have no potential conflicts of interest with respect to the research, authorship, or publication of this article.

REFERENCES

1. Jones CP. Confronting institutionalized racism. *Phylon*. 2002;50(1/2):7–22. https://doi.org/10.2307/4149999
2. Gee GC, Ford CL. Structural racism and health inequities: old issues, new directions. *Du Bois Rev*. 2011;8(1):115–132. https://doi.org/10.1017/s1742058x11000130
3. Boyd R, Lindo E, Weeks L, McLemore M. On racism: a new standard for publishing on racial health inequities. *Health Affairs Forefront Blog*. July 2, 2020. Available at: https://www.healthaffairs.org/do/10.1377/forefront.20200630.939347. Accessed December 12, 2025.
4. Howe CJ, Bailey ZD, Raifman JR, Jackson JW. Recommendations for using causal diagrams to study racial health disparities. *Am J Epidemiol*. 2022;191(12):1981–1989. https://doi.org/10.1093/aje/kwac140
5. Duncan AF, Montoya-Williams D. Recommendations for reporting research about racial disparities in medical and scientific journals. *JAMA Pediatr*. 2024;178(3):221–224. https://doi.org/10.1001/jamapediatrics.2023.5718
6. National Academies of Sciences, Engineering, and Medicine. *Rethinking Race and Ethnicity in Biomedical Research*. The National Academies Press. 2025. Available at: https://www.nationalacademies.org/projects/HMD-HSP-22-14/publication/27913. Accessed December 12, 2025.
7. Bailey ZD, Krieger N, Agénor M, Graves J, Linos N, Bassett MT. Structural racism and health inequities in the USA: evidence and interventions. *Lancet*. 2017;389(10077):1453–1463. https://doi.org/10.1016/s0140-6736(17)30569-x
8. Braveman PA, Arkin E, Proctor D, Kauh T, Holm N. Systemic and structural racism: definitions, examples, health damages, and approaches to dismantling. *Health Aff (Millwood)*. 2022;41(2):171–178. https://doi.org/10.1377/hlthaff.2021.01394
9. Lee C. "Race" and "ethnicity" in biomedical research: how do scientists construct and explain differences in health? *Soc Sci Med*. 2009;68(6):1183–1190. https://doi.org/10.1016/j.socscimed.2008.12.036
10. Orakwue K, Hing AK, Chantarat T, et al. The C2DREAM framework: investigating the structural mechanisms undergirding racial health inequities. *J Clin Transl Sci*. 2024;8(1):e80. https://doi.org/10.1017/cts.2024.518
11. Vyas DA, Eisenstein LG, Jones DS. Hidden in plain sight—reconsidering the use of race correction in clinical algorithms. *N Engl J Med*. 2020;383(9):874–882. https://doi.org/10.1056/NEJMms2004740
12. Nazer LH, Zatarah R, Waldrip S, et al. Bias in artificial intelligence algorithms and recommendations for mitigation. *PLOS Digit Health*. 2023;2(6):e0000278. https://doi.org/10.1371/journal.pdig.0000278

Evidentiary Pragmatism in Transgender Health Care

Florence Ashley, BCL/JD, LLM (Bioeth), SJD

ABOUT THE AUTHOR

Florence Ashley is with the Faculty of Law and John Dossetor Health Ethics Centre, University of Alberta, Edmonton, AB, Canada.

AJPH March 2026, Vol. 116, No. 3

In early 2025, the White House issued an executive order prohibiting funding for gender-affirming health care for minors, including puberty blockers and hormone therapy. Calling for the end of "reliance on junk science," the order echoed claims that the evidence base on gender-affirming health care is of low quality and thus insufficient to justify offering it.[1,2]

Medicine often proceeds from imperfect evidence. The majority of medical practices, including those recommended in World Health Organization guidelines, are predicated on low- or very low–quality evidence.[3–6] This is doubly true in the context of child and adolescent medicine.[7] Gender-affirming health care is often subject to greater scrutiny than equivalent interventions in other populations.[8] Setting aside the question of whether it is accurate to describe the evidence base of gender-affirming health care as low quality, more evidence is always welcome, and clinicians offering gender-affirming health care have been at the forefront of the quest to expand our knowledge of how to best care for transgender people. However, this does not mean that clinical decision-making and policy should ignore the best available evidence while waiting for better evidence.

Opposition to gender-affirming health care on evidentiary grounds has placed transgender communities in a catch-22. Observational studies that are relatively short are considered too weak to support access to gender-affirming health care, whereas longer-term observational studies are discounted for having significant participant attrition or being "too old" and therefore not representing the current clinical population.[9] As for randomized controlled trials, they do not offer a reliable alternative because of expected mass withdrawal from the control arm as well as noncompliance, crossover, response bias, and ethical concerns.[10,11] There is, it seems, no way to satisfy critics of gender-affirming health care.

This catch-22 has only been aggravated by Donald Trump's presidential administration, which has banned research on gender-affirming health care for minors, removed gender identity from Centers for Disease Control and Prevention data, and slashed National Institutes of Health funding. Even if alternative sources of funding are found, conservative attacks, harassment, and federal- and state-level bans on gender-affirming health care are making it extremely difficult, if not impossible, to study. Studying gender-affirming health care requires funding, institutional support, and the ability to offer the studied interventions. The Trump administration's attacks on gender-affirming care will have worldwide repercussions. The United States is the largest funder of research in the world and produces nearly half the publications on transgender health care worldwide.[12] Given the current rise in antitrans bills across the world, the monumental reduction in transgender health research in the United States will have global ramifications and may contribute to the banning of gender-affirming health care in other countries.

Access to interventions should not be predicated on unreasonable evidentiary expectations. It would be a perversion of science if beneficial—or at least harmless—interventions were impossible to ever be offered because the requested strength of evidence could not realistically be achieved. For instance, asking for randomized controlled trials for all interventions would be inappropriate because not all questions can realistically be studied using the methodology.[13] Similarly, minimal participant attrition may not be realistic in a long-term observational study.

The rights of marginalized groups should not depend on unrealistic, unreasonable, or impossible to meet evidentiary standards. Nor should they depend on evidentiary standards that the group has no reasonable opportunity to meet—which occurs when research is prohibited, funding is severely restricted, or funding is allocated unfairly. This is a matter of health policy, ethics, and human rights. As a matter of health policy, truly beneficial care should never be placed out of reach. As a matter of ethics and human rights, placing unrealistic demands on marginalized groups belies the bioethical principle of justice as well as the promise of human rights.

Given the foregoing, the principle of evidentiary pragmatism should be recognized as a core component of evidence evaluation, clinical decision-making, and policymaking. Evidentiary pragmatism requires that actionable conclusions be shaped by the levels of evidence that are reasonably achievable. A level of evidence is reasonably achievable when we can realistically design and complete a study that, if the hypothesis is true, can be expected to meet that evidentiary standard. For example, high-quality evidence could not be achieved through a randomized controlled trial if we can reasonably expect such trials to effectively become observational studies because of asymmetrical withdrawal, or if they would be fundamentally flawed by severe systematic bias—whether or not that bias is recognized in the grading scheme.

Authors should carefully explain which levels of evidence are reasonably achievable and characterize their degree of achievability, including any significant barriers to feasibility. Factors that affect achievability include but are not limited to funding constraints, difficulty securing ethical approval, barriers to representative recruitment, likelihood of participant withdrawal, loss to follow-up, unmasking, noncompliance, and crossover, as well as any other factor that may lead to the level of evidence being downgraded or upgraded. To ensure the quality of an analysis, topic experts, such as clinicians, researchers, and members of the studied community, should be involved throughout the process because they can provide invaluable insights into the intervention and population under study as well as probable participant behavior.

When reviewing scientific evidence and generating clinical or policy recommendations, studies should be assessed relative to both the highest reasonably achievable level of evidence and the degree to which that level is attainable. Conclusions and recommendations should follow the principles (1) that evidence quality must be judged in relation to what is reasonably achievable, rather than the highest possible evidentiary level; and (2) that interventions should not depend on evidence standards that cannot realistically be met. Although this should be done in all evidence evaluation, it is especially important when applying frameworks that formalize levels of evidence, such as GRADE (the Grading of Recommendations Assessment, Development and Evaluation framework), which systematizes the appraisal of evidence quality and recommendation strength.

When moderate-quality evidence is the highest reasonably achievable standard, consistent low-quality evidence should be weighed similarly to consistent moderate-quality evidence when high-quality evidence is achievable. When only low- or moderate-quality evidence is reasonably feasible, consistent low-quality evidence should typically be sufficient to ground a clinical recommendation or policy, the content of which should be informed by what the evidence shows. This approach aligns with current practice. Under the GRADE framework, a strong recommendation is one that should generally be followed because the expected benefits clearly outweigh the harms, even when the underlying evidence is of low quality. More than half of World Health Organization strong recommendations are based on low- or very low–quality evidence, and the American Academy of Pediatrics expressly recognizes cases in which "high-quality studies have not been performed and are unlikely ever to be performed,"[14(p34)] yet strong or moderate recommendations are warranted.[3,15] Groups developing clinical recommendations and policies must pay careful attention to the consistency, rigor, and comprehensiveness of reviews applying evidentiary pragmatism to mitigate the risk of biased conclusions drawn from cherry-picked lower-quality evidence.

Given the practical realities of transgender health, for which high-quality evidence is often unattainable and even moderate-quality evidence is difficult to produce, the predominance of low-quality evidence should not, by itself, justify restricting access—especially when that evidence is consistent.

The principles of medical ethics and human rights require us to not lose sight of the big picture when delving into highly technical evidentiary debates in which double standards abound. Respect for autonomy, beneficence, and justice are critical considerations in health care, as are the rights to equality and health. Although I have focused on transgender health care, the approach I have suggested may be beneficial to evidence assessment more generally, especially given the limits and weaknesses of evidence-based medicine in certain areas of research and the risk of double standards when controversial interventions are involved. Nobody's health care needs should be placed beyond proof. An inaccessible right is no right at all. AJPH

CORRESPONDENCE

Correspondence should be sent to Florence Ashley, University of Alberta Law Centre, 111 89 Ave NW, Edmonton, AB T6G 2H5 (e-mail: fashley@ualberta.ca). Reprints can be ordered at https://www.ajph.org by clicking the "Reprints" link.

PUBLICATION INFORMATION

Full Citation: Ashley F. Evidentiary pragmatism in transgender health care. *Am J Public Health*. 2026;116(3):304–306.

Acceptance Date: October 10, 2025.

DOI: https://doi.org/10.2105/AJPH.2025.308324

ORCID iD:

Florence Ashley https://orcid.org/0000-0001-9189-967X

CONFLICTS OF INTEREST

The author has no conflicts of interest to disclose.

REFERENCES

1. Cass H. *The Cass Review: Independent review of gender identity services for children and young people.* April 2024. Available at: https://cass.independent-review.uk/home/publications/final-report. Accessed November 18, 2025.
2. Miroshnychenko A, Ibrahim S, Roldan Y, et al. Gender affirming hormone therapy for individuals with gender dysphoria aged < 26 years: a systematic review and meta-analysis. *Arch Dis Child.* 2025;110(6):437–445. https://doi.org/10.1136/archdischild-2024-327921
3. Alexander PE, Bero L, Montori VM, et al. World Health Organization recommendations are often strong based on low confidence in effect estimates. *J Clin Epidemiol.* 2014;67(6):629–634. https://doi.org/10.1016/j.jclinepi.2013.09.020
4. Fleming PS, Koletsi D, Ioannidis JPA, Pandis N. High quality of the evidence for medical and other health-related interventions was uncommon in Cochrane systematic reviews. *J Clin Epidemiol.* 2016;78:34–42. https://doi.org/10.1016/j.jclinepi.2016.03.012
5. Howick J, Koletsi D, Pandis N, et al. The quality of evidence for medical interventions does not improve or worsen: a metaepidemiological study of Cochrane reviews. *J Clin Epidemiol.* 2020;126:154–159. https://doi.org/10.1016/j.jclinepi.2020.08.005
6. Howick J. Only one in ten medical treatments are backed by high-quality evidence. September 2, 2020. Available at: https://theconversation.com/only-one-in-ten-medical-treatments-are-backed-by-high-quality-evidence-145224. Accessed November 18, 2025.
7. Meng M, Zhou Q, Lei W, et al. Recommendations on off-label drug use in pediatric guidelines. *Front Pharmacol.* 2022;13:892574. https://doi.org/10.3389/fphar.2022.892574
8. Schall TE, Moses JD. Gender-affirming care for cisgender people. *Hastings Cent Rep.* 2023;53(3):15–24. https://doi.org/10.1002/hast.1486
9. Kingdon C, Stingelin-Giles N, Cass H. The Cass Review: distinguishing fact from fiction. *Am J Bioeth.* 2025;25(6):5–10. https://doi.org/10.1080/15265161.2025.2504397
10. Ashley F, Tordoff DM, Olson-Kennedy J, Restar AJ. Randomized-controlled trials are methodologically inappropriate in adolescent transgender healthcare. *Int J Transgend Health.* 2024;25(3):407–418. https://doi.org/10.1080/26895269.2023.2218357
11. Schall TE, Jaffe K, Moses JD. Roles of randomized controlled trials in establishing evidence-based gender-affirming care and advancing health equity. *AMA J Ethics.* 2024;26(9):E684–E689. https://doi.org/10.1001/amajethics.2024.684
12. Sweileh WM. Bibliometric analysis of peer-reviewed literature in transgender health (1900–2017). *BMC Int Health Hum Rights.* 2018;18(1):16. https://doi.org/10.1186/s12914-018-0155-5
13. Frieden TR. Evidence for health decision making—beyond randomized, controlled trials. *N Engl J Med.* 2017;377(5):465–475. https://doi.org/10.1056/NEJMra1614394
14. Alvarez F, Franklin W, Gleeson S. Evidence-based clinical practice guidelines: development and implementation manual. November 20, 2019. Available at: https://downloads.aap.org/DOCCSA/CPGManual20190628.pdf. Accessed November 18, 2025.
15. Matheny Antommaria AH, Kelleher M, Peterson RJ. Quality of evidence and strength of recommendations in American Academy of Pediatrics' guidelines. *Pediatrics.* 2025;155(4):e2024067836. https://doi.org/10.1542/peds.2024-067836

A Venue-Based Approach to Asymptomatic Mpox Screening and Doxy-PEP Provision: From Outbreak to Outreach, San Francisco, California, 2023–2024

Caitlin A. Contag, MD, Zachary T. Renfro, BS, Adi Xiyal Mukund, MD, PhD, Meg Quint, BS, Shannon Amitin, Vivian Levy, MD, Phillip L. Hammack, PhD, Benjamin A. Pinsky, MD, PhD, and Benjamin Laniakea, MD

The 2022 global outbreak of clade IIb mpox disproportionately impacted lesbian, gay, bisexual, transgender, and queer (LGBTQ+) communities and highlighted issues of stigma, access to health care, and health care–associated trauma. Together with LGBTQ+ community partners, our research team implemented venue-based mpox virus and antibody testing. In response to feedback from our community partners, this effort evolved to include broader elements of sexual health services, including distribution of prescriptions for doxycycline postexposure prophylaxis. *(Am J Public Health.* 2026;116(3):307–311. https://doi.org/10.2105/AJPH.2025.308309)

AJPH March 2026, Vol. 116, No. 3

From 2023 to 2024, our research team collaborated with lesbian, gay, bisexual, transgender, and queer (LGBTQ+) community partners to implement mpox research at sex-positive events. This article describes our approach to conducting research in this setting, as well as opportunities and challenges that arose during the process.

INTERVENTION AND IMPLEMENTATION

The primary aim of our study was to characterize the prevalence of asymptomatic or minimally symptomatic mpox virus (MPXV) infection in a highly exposed population in San Francisco, California. We analyzed self-collected oropharyngeal swab samples for the presence of MPXV nucleic acid by polymerase chain reaction (PCR). Second, we aimed to validate an MPXV antibody assay in blood and saliva and to characterize the antibody response to MPXV.

Our third aim was to be culturally competent liaisons between the biomedical and LGBTQ+ communities and to disseminate high-quality information about mpox without reinforcing shame or stigma around queer sex. By attending community events longitudinally and staying after sample collection ended, we meaningfully engaged with community members on diverse sexual health topics. In response to community feedback, we added a fourth aim: to offer information about, and free access to, doxycycline postexposure prophylaxis (doxy-PEP) prescriptions.

PLACE, TIME, AND PERSONS

This study took place over six events in several venues located throughout San Francisco from June 2023 to September 2024. Organized by and for queer communities, these events are central to the Bay Area kink scene and act as key facilitators of hookup culture. Notably, most events featured paid performers who consider themselves sex workers. Any individual aged 18 years or older could consent to study participation. Overall, we enrolled 231 individuals in this study (age range = 18–74 years) and wrote 104 doxy-PEP prescriptions (100 mg; n = 30; no refills). Study workflow is described in Figure 1. Individuals were eligible for doxy-PEP if they were men who have sex with men (MSM) or

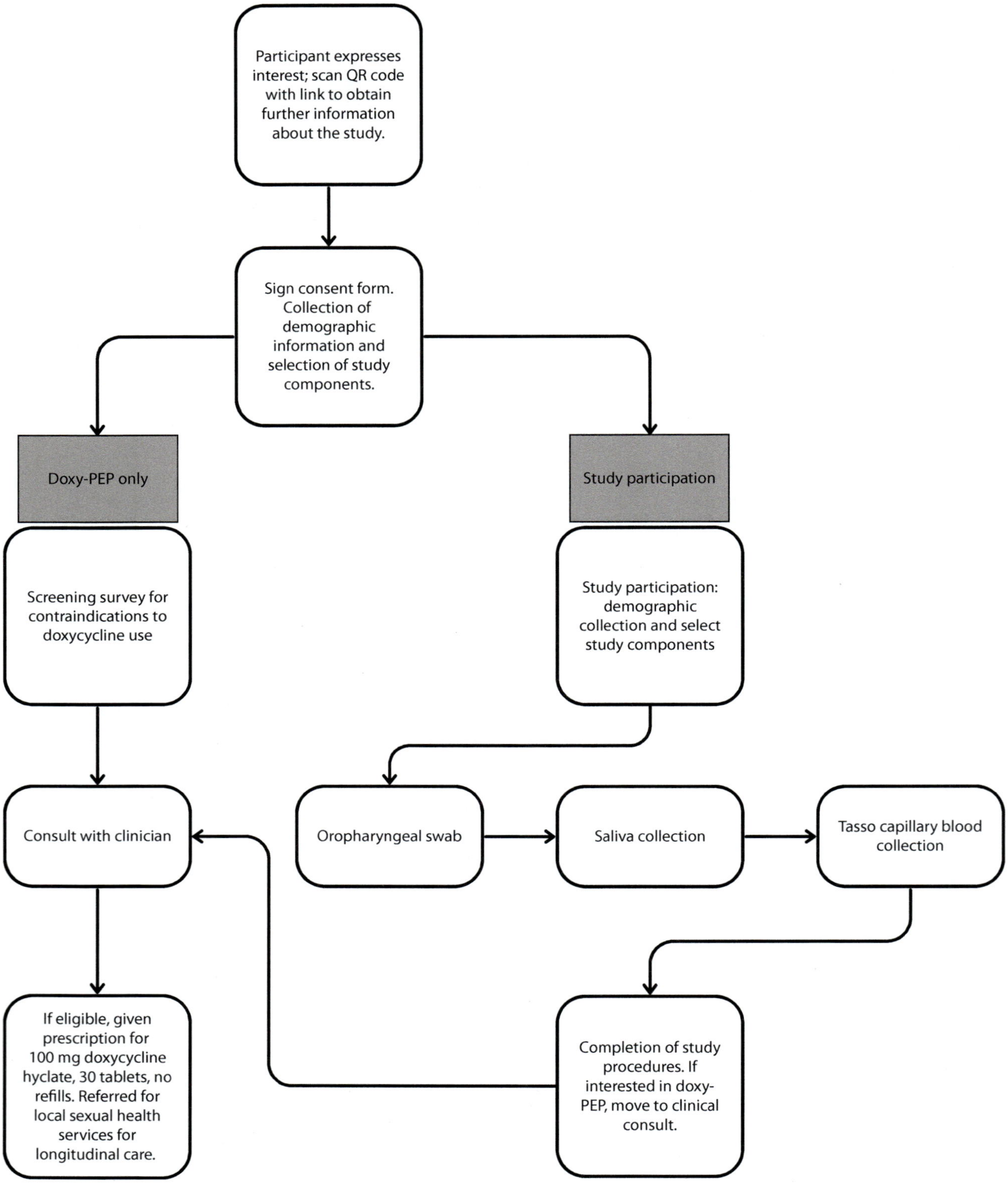

FIGURE 1— Mobile Venue-Based Testing Workflow for Mpox Virus and Antibody Testing at LGBTQ+ Sex-Positive Events: San Francisco, CA, 2023–2024

Note. doxy-PEP = doxycycline postexposure prophylaxis; LGBTQ+ = lesbian, gay, bisexual, transgender, and queer. If interested in both doxy-PEP and study participation, demographic collection and doxy-PEP screening were conducted at the same time.

transgender and did not report any contraindications to doxycycline. Most participants self-identified as male (206/231) and gay (175/231), bisexual (33/231), or queer (20/231). The majority of participants self-identified as White (87/140), followed by Hispanic (29/140), Asian (18/140), Black or African American (11/140), or Indigenous or Native American (4/140). Ninety-one participants declined to provide race/ethnicity data. Outcome data were not collected from those prescribed doxy-PEP. In the future, we will consider postprescription surveys to describe prescription fill rate and barriers to use.

PURPOSE

The 2022 clade IIb mpox outbreak was the largest ever, with more than 100 000 infections reported in nearly 100 nonendemic nations and was primarily driven through sexual networks of MSM and transgender persons. In the United States, a significant percentage of people diagnosed with mpox had HIV and belonged to racial or ethnic minority populations.[1–4] The clinical presentation of MPXV infection differed from previous outbreaks, with symptoms primarily localized to the anogenital and oropharyngeal areas.[3] Furthermore, the prevalence of asymptomatic MPXV infection was greater than previously reported.[5–7] Despite the efficacy of vaccination in preventing MPXV infection, the mucosal antibody response to MPXV has been incompletely characterized. As such, we aimed to describe the prevalence of asymptomatic MPXV infection in a highly exposed cohort of individuals, to validate an MPXV antibody assay in saliva and blood, and to characterize the serological response to infection or vaccination.

Throughout this outbreak, a major challenge has been effectively communicating evolving knowledge about MPXV, especially spread through sexual transmission, without propagating shame or stigma about LGBTQ+ communities or queer sex. This is compounded by lower levels of access to medical care and the historical mistreatment of LGBTQ+ communities by the biomedical establishment.[8–10] Many individuals in our research team are themselves LGBTQ+ and have experienced these challenges firsthand. To us, the mpox outbreak was not an abstract public health issue but, rather, the cause of significant distress and anxiety in our communities. Furthermore, we believe that the widespread dissemination of evidence-based information is a prerequisite for genuine sexual empowerment and bodily autonomy. As a largely queer research team with extensive experience in clinical infectious disease and epidemiology, we felt uniquely qualified to both generate and disseminate new knowledge to the communities to which we belong.

During this project, several studies were published showing the efficacy of doxy-PEP in preventing infection with bacterial sexually transmitted infections (STIs) in MSM.[11,12] In response to community feedback and to reach those with limited health care access, we implemented free counseling and prescription of doxy-PEP to eligible individuals, irrespective of participation in our study.

EVALUATION AND ADVERSE EFFECTS

Overall, we received an enthusiastic welcome from both organizers and the community at venues that participated. We enrolled 231 individuals in this study, from whom we collected 128 oropharyngeal swab samples for orthopoxvirus PCR testing, and 194 saliva samples and 39 blood samples for MPXV antibody testing (Stanford Clinical Virology Laboratory, Stanford, California; Orthopoxvirus IgG Panel, Meso Scale Diagnostics, Rockville, Maryland). One swab sample was positive for MPXV nucleic acid; this individual was referred for confirmatory diagnostic testing. Mpox incidence in California peaked between July 2022 and January 2023; the low sample positivity rate reflects this decline during the study period and suggests that asymptomatic infection was uncommon in this cohort.[13] Antibody assay validation and analysis are ongoing. Uptake of doxy-PEP prescribing was high, with 104 persons accepting written prescriptions over the three events where it was offered. During this pilot project, we did not offer baseline STI screening; in future work, we would consider offering point-of-care testing. Individuals were counseled that doxy-PEP is not considered treatment of existing STIs and were referred to local sexual health services.

In addition, throughout this project, we engaged with hundreds of individuals who did not formally participate in our study but did want to discuss aspects of sexual health. Our conversations were wide ranging, including updates on the mpox outbreak and current recommendations about reducing risk of infection, the prevalence and meaning of asymptomatic MPXV infection, and the effectiveness of vaccination against MPXV. We also partook in many conversations about doxy-PEP, including what evidence supports its use, who is likely to benefit from doxy-PEP, and comparing the benefit of incident STI prevention in high-risk individuals against concerns about antibiotic resistance.

Our study highlights the feasibility of a venue-based approach both for community-based monitoring of

AJPH March 2026, Vol. 116, No. 3

emerging pathogens and for supporting the sexual health and autonomy of LGBTQ+ communities (as evidenced by the high uptake of free doxy-PEP prescribing). San Francisco, with a large LGBTQ+ population and vibrant nightlife scene, is well suited for this type of intervention. This approach would likely be applicable in other locations, with modifications for local context including social determinants of health, religiosity, and perceived safety of LGBTQ+ spaces. Given early and widespread adoption of doxy-PEP in San Francisco, a venue-based approach may be more effective for doxy-PEP dissemination elsewhere. In discussions with community members and event organizers, no adverse effects of our intervention were reported to us.

SUSTAINABILITY

Mobile venue-based screening is a sustainable approach both to epidemiological surveys investigating emerging infectious diseases in high-risk populations and to promoting the sexual health of LGBTQ+ communities. Given the episodic nature of infectious disease outbreaks, it is unnecessary to continue operations longitudinally. However, once initial infrastructure has been established, it is remarkably easy to deploy venue-based screening; if a resurgence of mpox occurs, our team is well poised to reestablish our mobile testing operations within days.

The infrastructure required for this approach is cheap and relatively limited, fitting into the trunk of a vehicle and requiring less than half an hour for setup (Table 1). Venue-based screening can focus on particular populations at high risk for a particular infection, increasing the effectiveness of this approach. While our project focused on venues hosting kink and sex-positive LGBTQ+ events where people could meet new sexual partners, this approach can be adapted for different contexts tailored to relevant communities with epidemiological risk factors.[14,15] Furthermore, our focus on events celebrating queer sex and attended by sex workers positioned us well to effectively distribute doxy-PEP to a population that is likely to benefit from this service. Lastly, by longitudinally attending events serving the community we work in, biomedical researchers and public health officials can establish trusting connections with community members and provide evidence-based counseling about sexual health. Moreover, by centering queer voices and adapting our interventions to their expressed needs, our approach provides a pathway to rebuild the trust many LGBTQ+ communities have lost in the biomedical establishment.

TABLE 1— Equipment Used for Venue-Based Mobile Mpox Virus and Antibody Testing at LGBTQ+ Sex-Positive Events: San Francisco, CA, 2023–2024

Equipment	Amount
Basic supplies	
Folding table, 6 × 2.5 feet	1
Tablecloth	1
Illuminated sign	1
Hanging "virus" lights	5
Laminated consent form QR code	3
Styrofoam cooler	1
Tube rack	3
Timer	2
Masking tape	1
Physical prescription pad	2
Testing supplies	
Latex gloves: small, medium, large	1 each
Medium trash bag	1
Aptima multitest swab specimen kit	150
Tasso+ blood collection device	50
Saliva collection kit	100
Disposables	
Gum, individually wrapped	400
Temporary tattoos	200
Light-up "virus" necklaces	50
Glow necklaces with connectors	100
Candy, individually wrapped	100

Note. LGBTQ+ = lesbian, gay, bisexual, transgender, and queer.

PUBLIC HEALTH SIGNIFICANCE

Infectious disease surveillance is a cornerstone of public health and allows us to make better-informed decisions with limited resources. Traditional infectious disease surveillance relies heavily on laboratory and clinician-reported data, which are resource intensive and experience significant time delays. This is particularly problematic for emerging infections or when considering populations that experience significant barriers to obtaining clinical care.

Through establishing a venue-based approach to MPXV screening, we effectively addressed both issues. By meeting individuals in the communities in which they live, work, and play, we were able not only to characterize the epidemiology of MPXV in San Francisco but also to increase community awareness of and knowledge about MPXV, tailored to unique individual concerns. An integral component of sexual autonomy is access to relevant health information and the freedom to act upon that information as one desires. Through framing our intervention as a celebration of queer sex and a desire to support queer sexual autonomy, we were able to disseminate information about MPXV to community members without propagating shame or stigma. AJPH

ABOUT THE AUTHORS

Caitlin A. Contag is with the Department of Pulmonary, Allergy, and Critical Care Medicine at Stanford University School of Medicine, Stanford, CA. Zachary T. Renfro and Meg Quint are dual MD and MS students at the Stanford University School of Medicine. Adi Xiyal Mukund was a dual MD and PhD student at the Stanford University School of Medicine at the time of this study. Shannon Amitin is with QT Cruising, San Francisco. Vivian Levy is with San Mateo Medical Center, San Mateo, CA. Phillip L. Hammack is with the University of California, Santa Cruz. Benjamin A. Pinsky is with the Clinical Virology Laboratory for Stanford Health Care, Stanford. Benjamin Laniakea is with the Stanford LGBTQ+ Adult Clinical Program, Stanford University School of Medicine.

CORRESPONDENCE

Correspondence should be sent to Zachary T. Renfro, 291 Campus Dr, Stanford, CA 94305 (e-mail: ztrenfro@stanford.edu). Reprints can be ordered at https://www.ajph.org by clicking the "Reprints" link.

PUBLICATION INFORMATION

Full Citation: Contag CA, Renfro ZT, Mukund AX, et al. A venue-based approach to asymptomatic mpox screening and doxy-PEP provision: from outbreak to outreach, San Francisco, California, 2023–2024. *Am J Public Health*. 2026;116(3): 307–311.

Acceptance Date: October 1, 2025.

DOI: https://doi.org/10.2105/AJPH.2025.308309

ORCID iDs:

Zachary T. Renfro https://orcid.org/0000-0002-9927-4452

Adi Xiyal Mukund https://orcid.org/0000-0003-2752-1458

Shannon Amitin https://orcid.org/0009-0007-4468-5717

Vivian Levy https://orcid.org/0009-0005-6613-1948

Phillip L. Hammack https://orcid.org/0000-0003-2203-858X

CONTRIBUTORS

C. A. Contag and Z. T. Renfro were co-first authors; they contributed equally to this work and were jointly responsible for project conceptualization, organization with community groups, data acquisition and analysis, and article preparation. A. X. Mukund and M. Quint contributed to organization with community groups and data acquisition. S. Amitin and P. L. Hammack contributed to organizing with community partners and communicating feedback from community members. V. Levy and B. Laniakea contributed to project design and data acquisition. B. A. Pinsky contributed to project design and data analysis. All authors reviewed and offered feedback on the article before publication.

ACKNOWLEDGMENTS

This work was funded with intramural research funds from the Stanford University School of Medicine.

We would like to thank Yaowei Deng, Fumiko Yamamoto, and Müge Kalaycıoğlu for their dedication and contributions to this project. In addition, we owe a debt of gratitude to the participants in our research who have welcomed us, engaged us, and challenged us. They are our invaluable teachers.

CONFLICTS OF INTEREST

The authors have no conflicts of interest, financial or otherwise, to disclose.

HUMAN PARTICIPANT PROTECTION

This project was approved by the Stanford University School of Medicine institutional review board.

REFERENCES

1. Angelo KM, Smith T, Camprubí-Ferrer D, GeoSentinel Network Collaborators, et al. Epidemiological and clinical characteristics of patients with monkeypox in the GeoSentinel Network: a cross-sectional study. *Lancet Infect Dis*. 2023;23(2):196–206. https://doi.org/10.1016/S1473-3099(22)00651-X
2. Vusirikala A, Charles H, Balasegaram S, et al. Epidemiology of early monkeypox virus transmission in sexual networks of gay and bisexual men, England, 2022. *Emerg Infect Dis*. 2022;28(10):2082–2086. https://doi.org/10.3201/eid2810.220960
3. Titanji BK, Hazra A, Zucker J. Mpox clinical presentation, diagnostic approaches, and treatment strategies: a review. *JAMA*. 2024;332(19):1652–1662. https://doi.org/10.1001/jama.2024.21091
4. Kava CM, Rohraff DM, Wallace B, et al. Epidemiologic features of the monkeypox outbreak and the public health response—United States, May 17–October 6, 2022. *MMWR Morb Mortal Wkly Rep*. 2022;71(45):1449–1456. https://doi.org/10.15585/mmwr.mm7145a4
5. Contag CA, Lu J, Renfro ZT, et al. Retrospective screening of clinical samples for monkeypox virus DNA, California, USA, 2022. *Emerg Infect Dis*. 2023;29(4):848–850. https://doi.org/10.3201/eid2904.221576
6. Contag CA, Renfro ZT, Lu J, et al. Prevalence of mpox (monkeypox) in patients undergoing STI screening in northern California, April–September 2022. *J Clin Virol*. 2023;164:105493. https://doi.org/10.1016/j.jcv.2023.105493
7. De Baetselier I, Van Dijck C, Kenyon C, ITM Monkeypox study group, et al. Retrospective detection of asymptomatic monkeypox virus infections among male sexual health clinic attendees in Belgium. *Nat Med*. 2022;28(11):2288–2292. https://doi.org/10.1038/s41591-022-02004-w
8. Casey LS, Reisner SL, Findling MG, et al. Discrimination in the United States: experiences of lesbian, gay, bisexual, transgender, and queer Americans. *Health Serv Res*. 2019;54(suppl 2):1454–1466. https://doi.org/10.1111/1475-6773.13229
9. Eaton LA, Driffin DD, Kegler C, et al. The role of stigma and medical mistrust in the routine health care engagement of Black men who have sex with men. *Am J Public Health*. 2015;105(2):e75–e82. https://doi.org/10.2105/AJPH.2014.302322
10. Goldenberg T, Jadwin-Cakmak L, Popoff E, Reisner SL, Campbell BA, Harper GW. Stigma, gender affirmation, and primary healthcare use among Black transgender youth. *J Adolesc Health*. 2019;65(4):483–490. https://doi.org/10.1016/j.jadohealth.2019.04.029
11. Luetkemeyer AF, Donnell D, Dombrowski JC, DoxyPEP Study Team, et al. Postexposure doxycycline to prevent bacterial sexually transmitted enfections. *N Engl J Med*. 2023;388(14):1296–1306. https://doi.org/10.1056/NEJMoa2211934
12. Bolan RK, Beymer MR, Weiss RE, Flynn RP, Leibowitz AA, Klausner JD. Doxycycline prophylaxis to reduce incident syphilis among HIV-infected men who have sex with men who continue to engage in high-risk sex: a randomized, controlled pilot study. *Sex Transm Dis*. 2015;42(2):98–103. https://doi.org/10.1097/OLQ.0000000000000216
13. California Department of Public Health, Division of Communicable Disease Control. MPOX data in California. Available at: https://www.cdph.ca.gov/Programs/CID/DCDC/Pages/Mpox-Data.aspx. Accessed March 12, 2025.
14. Patel RR, Luke DA, Proctor EK, et al. Sex venue-based network analysis to identify HIV prevention dissemination targets for men who have sex with men. *LGBT Health*. 2018;5(1):78–85. https://doi.org/10.1089/lgbt.2017.0018
15. Ott MA, Campbell J, Imburgia TM, Yang Z, Tu W, Auerswald CL. Community engagement and venue-based sampling in adolescent male sexually transmitted infection prevention research. *J Adolesc Health*. 2018;62(3 suppl):S58–S64. https://doi.org/10.1016/j.jadohealth.2017.10.002

Umoja Health: Building Community Coalitions to Achieve Health Equity From COVID-19 to Cancer

Kim F. Rhoads, MD, MS, MPH, Eva N. Pardo, MPH, Salustiano Ribeiro, MSc, Ghilamichael Andemeskel, Monique LeSarre, PsyD, Noha Aboelata, MD, Lisa M. Tealer, Damon Francis, MD, Zhonnet Harper, Kala M. Mehta, DSc, MPH, Jonathan D. Fuchs, MD, MPH, and Kimi Watkins-Tartt

Umoja Health (UH) is a community-led approach to address long-standing disparities in health. UH was founded in 2020 at the request of members of the University of California, San Francisco Cancer Center Community Advisory Board. UH started with a focus on COVID-19 testing in San Francisco Bay Area Black/African American communities and evolved to address chronic disease and cancer in diverse communities. We detail UH's approach to addressing the separation between public health and health care, highlighting the coalition's effects on local health equity. (*Am J Public Health*. 2026;116(3):312–316. https://doi.org/10.2105/AJPH.2025.308322)

AJPH March 2026, Vol. 116, No. 3

The COVID-19 pandemic exposed the detrimental effects of the separation of public health from health care in the United States. This historical disconnect, which slows progress toward health equity, is often met with interventions that aim to build a proverbial bridge to close the gap between institutions and communities. Umoja Health (UH), by contrast, is a community-led approach to achieving health equity by building a multisectoral coalition to operate in and fill, rather than bridge, the gap. The UH coalition connected financial and human resources at large health care institutions to community-based public health efforts to reduce the burden of COVID-19. Over time, UH evolved to address chronic disease and cancer.

INTERVENTION AND IMPLEMENTATION

The UH model started in early 2020. At that time, the University of California, San Francisco (UCSF) was providing free polymerase chain reaction COVID-19 testing in select San Francisco neighborhoods.[1,2] Long-standing UCSF Cancer Center Community Advisory Board[3] members from the Brotherhood of Elders Network[4] requested similar support for Black/African American communities in nearby Alameda County, a large (more than 500 000 residents) racially, ethnically, and socioeconomically diverse county in northern California.

The Brotherhood of Elders Network, an influential intergenerational network of men of African descent, had convened the African American Response Circle health committee in response to the pandemic. Leadership and staff from the UCSF Cancer Center's Office of Community Engagement leveraged Brotherhood of Elders Network social capital to organize what eventually became the UH coalition. The coalition included Black/African American–focused community- and faith-based organizations, community advocates, the Alameda County Public Health Department (ACPHD), community health centers, for-profit business partners, municipal agencies, and staff of local elected officials.

UH used a three-pronged approach to build community coalitions with the capacity to achieve health equity. UH disseminated credible information, provided direct service delivery by and for the community, and supported workforce development to transform the future of public health and health care.

PLACE, TIME, AND PERSONS

Credible health information was disseminated via Zoom during the African American Response Circle health committee's weekly meetings. Local and state health department data dashboards informed partners and their networks about relevant trends in

COVID-19 transmission, hospitalizations, and deaths. The ACPHD epidemiology unit presented hyperlocal data by age, race/ethnicity, zip code, and census tract. Meetings provided updates on emerging discoveries, evolving recommendations for mitigation, and changes in Medicaid coverage when the public health emergency declaration lapsed. Participants also received information about funding, careers, and opportunities to participate in research.

UH partners determined locations for health services and pioneered community-led, no-barrier testing pop-ups in neighborhood settings. Locations ranged from the more typical (e.g., church parking lots and Black/African American–focused farmers' markets) to less traditional settings (e.g., public transit hubs, bodega store fronts, and street corners). Volunteer licensed providers from different, often competing health systems delivered clinical services and facilitated follow-up referrals. Pop-up events featured warm hand-offs to coalition partners with resources to address health-related social needs. Community members welcomed, registered, and surveyed participants to determine eligibility for cancer screening. The community call team provided wrap-around services (e.g., grocery delivery, scripted daily check-ins) for those testing positive for COVID-19. One health system purchased a van to transport supplies, many of which were acquired through philanthropic support.

Workforce development programming in 2021 responded to low vaccination rates among individuals 18 to 24 years of age.[5] UH partner organizations co-developed the UH Youth Mobilizers program and the six-week UH Workforce Summer Internship. The mobilizers, who were 18 to 30 years old, attended weekly meetings, conducted COVID-19 knowledge and awareness surveys, and developed COVID-19 messaging on social media channels. The interns learn about the separation of public health from health care and the impact of that gap on disparities. All UH workforce participants received college and career preparation and support.

In response to a subsequent request from community partners outside of Alameda County, UH expanded to San Mateo and San Francisco counties. The new coalitions increased UH reach in Latinx and Pacific Islander communities with expanded services to include colorectal and prostate cancer screening, flu vaccines, diabetes screening, and blood pressure monitoring.

PURPOSE

In the summer of 2020, COVID-19 testing in Alameda County was limited to a single Black-serving clinic system, Roots Community Health.[6] Although Roots offered low- to no-barrier testing, participants traveled from zip codes with high resources and low infection rates, while surrounding Black and Latino communities were less likely to partake. Centering community members in the design and delivery of the UH intervention transformed COVID-19 care uptake. In Swahili, Umoja means "unity." Umoja Health is a word play conveying the concept of being united in health. UH was the first program in Alameda County to meet people where they were and when they were there, linking them to resources available through the connections with UH coalition partners. Because of the UH success reaching key communities, ACPHD entrusted the coalition with a vaccine supply (managed by commercial partner Bay Area Phlebotomy Lab Services) for distribution.

EVALUATION AND ADVERSE EFFECTS

The UH logic model (Figure 1) highlights the immediate and intermediate effects of the UH intervention on health outcomes and the San Francisco Bay Area health ecosystem. To date, the UH coalition has convened more than 250 Zoom meetings across three counties. The network of partners includes more than 100 faith- and community-based organizations that provide services for Black/African American, Latinx, and Pacific Islander individuals along with three public health departments, five Federally Qualified Health Centers, four competing health systems, one school district, and a handful of staff of local elected officials.

As a direct result of funding opportunities introduced in UH meetings and technical assistance provided by coalition members with grant writing experience, UH partners secured more than $2.5 million in contracts and grants to support pandemic and cancer control efforts between 2020 and 2023. Coalition members developed messaging campaigns promoting masking, Medicaid reenrollment, cancer screening, and early detection. Messages were placed on public transportation, on freeway billboards, and in radio public service announcements, garnering more than 30 million impressions.

UH facilitated more than 500 pop-up events and administered and distributed more than 10 000 COVID tests and 7000 COVID and other vaccinations. In addition, the program completed 1233 chronic disease screenings and 179 cancer screenings and navigated more than 38 Bay Area residents into cancer care, leveraging resources across the network.

UH trained 72 youth mobilizers and interns, 80% from groups underrepresented in medicine. Table 1 details their

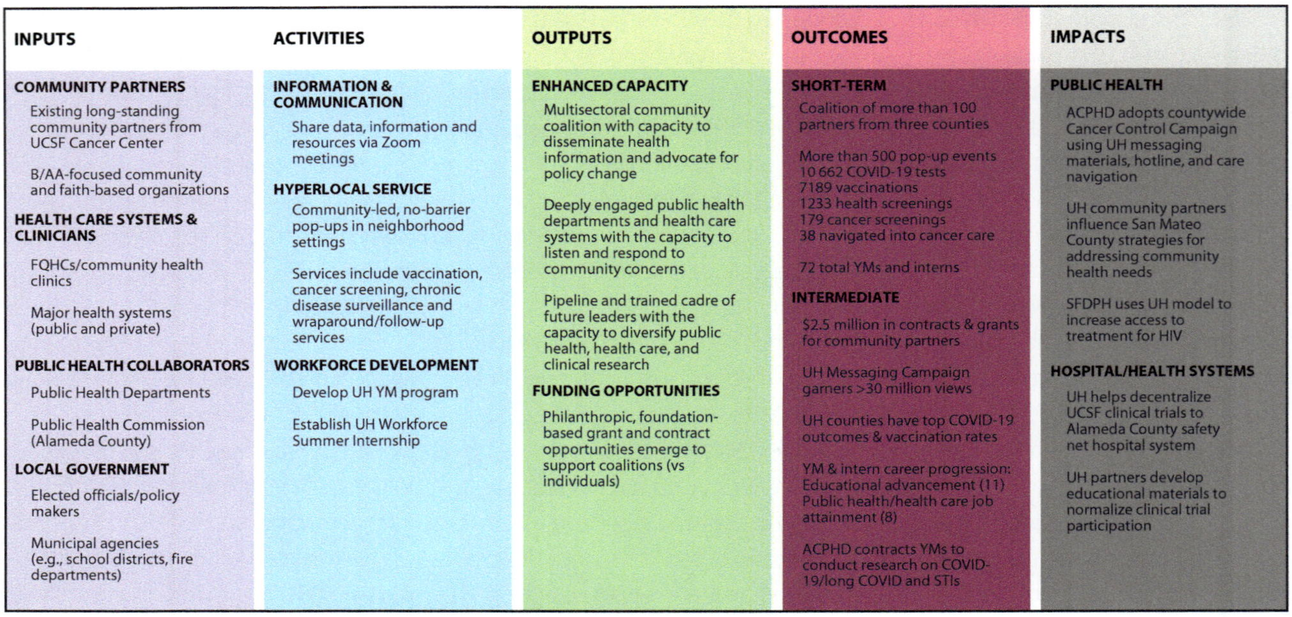

FIGURE 1— Umoja Health Logic Model: California, 2020–2025

Note. ACPHD = Alameda County Public Health Department; B/AA = Black/African American; FQHC = Federally Qualified Health Center; SFDPH = San Francisco Department of Public Health; STI = sexually transmitted infection; UCSF = University of California, San Francisco; UH = Umoja Health; YM = youth mobilizer.

sociodemographic characteristics and career progression. In 2024, ACPHD contracted the mobilizers to conduct survey-based research on COVID-19 and the drivers of sexually transmitted infections.

The UH model directly influenced ACPHD's implementation of vaccination points of distribution and development of contractual funding for community coalitions to mitigate COVID-19.[7] By fall 2023, the three UH counties (San Francisco, San Mateo, and Alameda) had the lowest COVID-19 death rates and the highest rates of vaccine uptake among Black/African American and Latinx populations in California's large counties.[8] Nationally, the city of Oakland, located in Alameda County, was recognized as a top performer on COVID-19 outcomes[9] despite a demographic profile that might predict otherwise.

TABLE 1— Demographic and Social Characteristics: Umoja Health Workforce Programs (California, 2021–2025)

	Youth Mobilizers	Summer Interns	Total
Age, mean ±SD	22 ±5.2	20 ±4.0	21 ±4.4
Male, no. (%)	12 (42.9)	6 (13.6)	18 (25.0)
Underrepresented in medicine, no. (%)	25 (89.3)	33 (75.0)	58 (80.6)
First-generation college, no. (%)	15 (53.6)	35 (79.6)	50 (69.4)
Educational career advancement,[a] no. (%)	7 (25.0)	4 (9.1)	11 (15.3)
Public health/health care job attainment,[b] no. (%)	4 (14.3)	4 (9.1)	8 (11.1)
Total, no.	28	44	72

Note. UCSF = University of California, San Francisco.
[a]Includes recent medical school application and matriculation, postbaccalaureate program enrollment, nursing entrance exam completion, master's/registered nursing program graduate, public health fellowship, and student lab researcher.
[b]Includes Alameda County Public Health Department public health analyst, certified medical assistant and phlebotomist, UCSF clinical research coordinator, UCSF data analyst, and certified community health worker.

SUSTAINABILITY

Existing foundational relationships fuel UH's success. UH was born out of two long-standing organizing bodies: the UCSF Cancer Center Community Advisory Board, founded in 2005, and the Brotherhood of Elders Network, founded in 2011.[3,4] The sustainability of UH is powered by public health department infrastructure and commitment to ongoing health messaging and promotion, coupled with local volunteer providers, community partners, and youth program participants. These tightly networked groups have increased capacity to engage health systems, advocate for change, and hold institutions accountable for addressing health disparities.

ACPHD is using youth mobilizer survey results and design ideas to guide sexually transmitted infection mitigation messages. Under the guidance of the Alameda County Public Health Commission, the department is exploring ways to incorporate UH cancer control efforts into ongoing community health functions. The San Mateo coalition continues to shape local public health strategies to address community health needs, and the San Francisco Department of Public Health replicated the UH model to increase access to HIV treatment.[10]

Current funding commitments support the sustainability of the UH coalition work. A $1.5 million grant from the Gilead Foundation is supporting decentralization of UCSF cancer clinical trials to the Alameda Health System, Alameda County's safety net hospital. Clinical research coordinators and community health educators hired from the UH coalition will play a pivotal role in demystifying the randomization process and normalizing the idea that clinical trials are an important and expected part of comprehensive cancer care. Additional industry funding will support the Youth Mobilizer and Summer Internship programs in 2026.

PUBLIC HEALTH SIGNIFICANCE

The gap between public health and health care can worsen health disparities. When COVID-19 threatened to exhaust local hospital resources, avoiding collapse required a public health intervention. The UH coalition model fills this gap by connecting novel material support (e.g., COVID-19 polymerase chain reaction testing, volunteer health providers, direct funding, donated vaccines) with human resources (youth workforce, community advocates) to energize public health efforts.

UH delivered better COVID-19 outcomes relative to other statewide and national localities. A similar outcome could be achieved in cancer disparities if public health departments support health messaging, disease prevention, and risk-reduction activities in collaboration with community partners and local health systems that can screen and navigate community members into care. UH is a scalable model for achieving health equity. Because the model has the potential to reduce the burden of disease and the costs of complex health care, commercial insurers and public payers should consider year-round investment in multisectoral coalitions such as Umoja Health. AJPH

ABOUT THE AUTHORS

Kim F. Rhoads, Eva N. Pardo, and Ghilamichael Andemeskel are with the Department of Epidemiology and Biostatistics and the Helen Diller Family Comprehensive Cancer Center, School of Medicine, University of California, San Francisco. Salustiano Ribeiro is with Bay Area Phlebotomy Lab Services, San Bruno, CA. Monique LeSarre is with the Berkeley-Oakland YWCA, Berkeley, CA. Noha Aboelata is with Roots Community Health, Oakland, CA. Lisa M. Tealer is with the Bay Area Community Health Advisory Council, Redwood City, CA. Damon Francis is with the Alameda Health System, Homeless Health Center, and Brotherhood of Elders Network, Oakland, CA. Zhonnet Harper is with the Alameda County Public Health Commission, San Leandro, CA. Kala M. Mehta is with the Department of Epidemiology and Biostatistics, School of Medicine, University of California, San Francisco. Jonathan D. Fuchs is with the San Francisco Department of Public Health, San Francisco, CA. Kimi Watkins-Tartt is with the Alameda County Public Health Department, San Leandro, CA.

CORRESPONDENCE

Correspondence should be sent to Kim F. Rhoads, MD, MS, MPH, Massey Comprehensive Cancer Center, Goodwin Research Laboratory, 401 College St, Richmond, VA 23298 (e-mail: kim.rhoads@vcuhealth.org). Reprints can be ordered at https://www.ajph.org by clicking the "Reprints" link.

PUBLICATION INFORMATION

Full Citation: Rhoads KF, Pardo EN, Ribeiro S, et al. Umoja Health: building community coalitions to achieve health equity from COVID-19 to cancer. *Am J Public Health*. 2026;116(3):312–316.

Acceptance Date: October 22, 2025.

DOI: https://doi.org/10.2105/AJPH.2025.308322

ORCID iDs:

Kim F. Rhoads https://orcid.org/0000-0002-2558-6509

Eva N. Pardo https://orcid.org/0009-0009-0466-1563

Salustiano Ribeiro https://orcid.org/0000-0002-7482-2336

Ghilamichael Andemeskel https://orcid.org/0009-0008-9231-0343

Damon Francis https://orcid.org/0009-0003-7713-7603

Zhonnet Harper https://orcid.org/0009-0001-6052-336X

CONTRIBUTORS

K. F. Rhoads, E. N. Pardo, S. Ribeiro, G. Andemeskel, and M. LeSarre drafted the article and made substantial contributions to the conception or design or acquisition, analysis, or interpretation of data. K. F. Rhoads, E. N. Pardo, L. M. Tealer, K. M. Mehta, J. D. Fuchs, and K. Watkins-Tartt drafted the article and made critical revisions and edits.

ACKNOWLEDGMENTS

This work was funded by the University of California, San Francisco (UCSF) School of Medicine, Kaiser Permanente, the Chan Zuckerberg Initiative, Life Sciences Cares Bay Area, the Crankstart Foundation, the Salesforce Corporation, the Alameda County Public Health Department and Healthcare Services

Agency, the San Francisco Department of Public Health, and community donors via Go Fund Me.

We acknowledge all of the Umoja Health partners, without whom this work would not have been possible: Laurie Long; Albert J. Burleson; Kevin Epps; Arnold Perkins, Former Chair of the UCSF Cancer Center Community Advisory Board; the Abundant Life Health Ministries Network of the UCSF Comprehensive Cancer Center; Anamatangi Polynesian Voices; 100 Black Men, Bay Area; 3rd Street Youth Center & Clinic; Acts Full Gospel Church of God in Christ; Adamika Village; Alameda County Public Health Department Community Assessment Planning and Evaluation Unit; Alameda Health Consortium; Arsola's House; Bay Area Black Nurses Association Inc.; Bay Nation Home Health; Bayview Child Health Center; Bayview YMCA; Bayview Senior Services; Belle Haven Action; Beth Eden Baptist Church; Bethlehem Lutheran Church; Bible Fellowship Missionary Baptist Church; Black Cultural Zone; BlackFullness; Building Opportunities for Self-Sufficiency; Both Sides of the Conversation; Brotherhood of Elders Network; California Prevention and Education Project; Center of Hope Community Church; Chan Zuckerberg Biohub; Charlotte Maxwell Clinic; Cheryl Ward Liberation Ministries; City of East Palo Alto; City of Menlo Park; City of Oakland; City of Palo Alto; City of Refuge Church; Community Health Center Network; County of San Mateo Office of Community Affairs; Cultura y Arte Nativa de las Americas; East Bay Getting to Zero; East Palo Alto Center for Community Media; Ecumenical Hunger Program; El Centro Bayview; UCSF-SFGH Family and Community Medicine Residents; Friends of Dr. Frank Staggers Sr.; Glad Tidings Church of God in Christ International; Global Communications, Education, and Art; Health Leads; Hip Hop For The People; Hoover Foster Resident Action Council; HOPE SF; House of Prayer Everywhere; Kafenia Peace Collective; Lifelong Medical Care; Marcus Foster Education Institute; Marie Harrison Community Foundation; Men of Influence; Black Men's Health Committee of the UCSF Comprehensive Cancer Center; MERCER Brotherhood; Mobile Attentive; Mr. Krispy Professional Barbershop; Neighborhood Baptist Church; Nuestra Casa of East Palo Alto; Oakland African American Chamber of Commerce; Oakland Fire Department; Oakland Frontline Healers; Oakland United School District; Office of (former) Alameda County Supervisor Keith Carson; Office of Alameda County Supervisor Nate Miley; Office of Menlo Park City Councilmember Cecilia Taylor; Office of (former) Oakland City Council District 3 Councilmember Carroll Fife; Office of (former) Oakland City Council District 6 Councilmember Loren Taylor; Office of (former) US Congresswoman Barbara Lee; Owning My Own Truth; Paradise Baptist Church; Peninsula Health Care District; Project Pet; Rafiki Coalition; Ravenswood City School District; Ravenswood Family Health Network; Realized Potential Inc.; Redwood City Together; Roots Community Health; Samaritan House; Samuel Merritt University Ethnic Health Institute; San Francisco Christian Center; San Francisco Department of Public Health; San Francisco Recreation and Parks; San Mateo County Health; San Mateo County Office of Education; Samoan Community Development Center; Serenity House; Stanford Health Care; Sutter Health; Together Toward Health, a program of the Public Health Institute; True Vine Ministries; UCSF Comprehensive Cancer Center; UCSF Roving Community Health Initiative; United in Love Inc.; Village Connect; WeHope; West Oakland Health Center; WISE Health SF; Women Organized to Respond to Life-threatening Diseases; Women's Cancer Resource Center; Young Community Developers; Youth Community Service; and Youth Uprising.

CONFLICTS OF INTEREST

The authors have no conflicts of interest to disclose.

HUMAN PARTICIPANT PROTECTION

No protocol approval was required because this research did not involve human participants.

REFERENCES

1. Fields J, Raul G, Marquez C, et al. Community-academic partnerships to address Covid-19 inequities: lessons from the San Francisco bay area. Available at: https://www.researchgate.net/publication/352863731_Community-Academic_Partnerships_to_Address_Covid-19_Inequities_Lessons_from_the_San_Francisco_Bay_Area. Accessed October 22, 2025.
2. United in Health. United in Health home page. Available at: https://unitedinhealth.org. Accessed October 22, 2025.
3. University of California, San Francisco Helen Diller Family Comprehensive Cancer Center. Community Advisory Board. Available at: https://cancer.ucsf.edu/community-engagement/cab. Accessed October 22, 2025.
4. Brotherhood of Elders Network. Brotherhood of Elders Network home page. Available at: https://brotherhoodofelders.net. Accessed October 22, 2025.
5. Diesel J, Sterrett N, Dasgupta S, et al. COVID-19 vaccination coverage among adults—United States, December 14, 2020–May 22, 2021. *MMWR Morb Mortal Wkly Rep.* 2021;70(25):922–927. https://doi.org/10.15585/mmwr.mm7025e1
6. Roots Community Health. Roots Community Health home page. Available at: https://rootscommunityhealth.org. Accessed October 22, 2025.
7. Alameda County Health Care Services Agency. Alameda County launches a new $12M initiative for the hyper-local phase of the COVID-19 response. Available at: https://covid-19.acgov.org/covid19-assets/docs/press/press-release-2021.06.03.pdf. Accessed October 22, 2025.
8. California Health and Human Services. California open data: COVID-19 time-series metrics by county and state. Available at: https://data.chhs.ca.gov/dataset/covid-19-time-series-metrics-by-county-and-state. Accessed April 18, 2022.
9. Linkhart D. Civic engagement success story: Alameda County, Oakland and COVID 19. Available at: https://www.nationalcivicleague.org/ncr-article/civic-engagement-success-story-alameda-county-oakland-and-covid-19. Accessed October 22, 2025.
10. Rafiki Coalition. Umoja Health access point. Available at: https://rafikicoalition.org/umoja-hap. Accessed October 22, 2025.

Post-*Dobbs* Era: Evolving Abortion Care Restrictions and Public Health Impact

Denys T. Lau, PhD, Jihong Liu, ScD, and Marian Moser Jones, PhD

ABOUT THE AUTHORS

Denys T. Lau is the AJPH *Editor-in-Chief and is with the Johns Hopkins University, Baltimore, MD; George Washington University, Washington, DC; and University of Illinois at Chicago. Jihong Liu is an* AJPH *Associate Editor and is with the Department of Epidemiology and Biostatistics, University of South Carolina, Columbia. Marian Moser Jones is an* AJPH *Associate Editor and is with the College of Public Health, The Ohio State University, Columbus.*

See also Abortion and Public Health Impact in Post-*Dobbs* Era, pp. 321–367.

The 2022 US Supreme Court ruling in *Dobbs v Jackson Women's Health Organization*, which overturned the federal constitutional right to abortion, quickly transformed abortion availability and access into a sharply contrasting state-based patchwork. By late 2025, 23 states had enacted near-total bans or strict gestational limits at 22 weeks or less that some argue may diverge from international standards for reproductive rights and care.[1,2] Meanwhile, the remaining states plus the District of Columbia maintained various levels of protections or enshrined abortion rights in state constitutions. Some protective states expanded services and enacted legislation shielding health care workers, including those providing reproductive health care to out-of-state residents, from out-of-state legal threats.[3] Emerging research now indicates that the shift in abortion laws to states has reshaped abortion care access and delivery, maternal and infant health outcomes, the health care workforce, and public health data monitoring systems.

Since *Dobbs*, abortion access and care have varied greatly by geography, as well as type and timing of care. Regional case studies have documented declines in abortion care seeking behaviors by women early in their pregnancies (e.g., volume of calls requesting financial assistance to offset abortion-related costs) and increases in care seeking at later gestational stages, perhaps because of legal restrictions, limited service availability, and travel and financial barriers.[4] Clinicians in restrictive states report delays in treating miscarriages, ectopic pregnancies, and cancer because of their own legal fears and confusion.[5] Meanwhile, medication abortions, especially via telehealth, have expanded under state "shield" laws that allow health care providers to legally mail abortion pills to patients in states with abortion bans. By 2023, medication abortions constituted 63% of all US abortions, with nearly 25% delivered via telemedicine in 2024.[6]

Pre-*Dobbs* data show that states with more restrictive abortion policies had higher maternal mortality rates than states with more protective policies.[7]

Continued on page 318...

HISTORY CORNER

39 YEARS AGO

Reproductive Mortality in the United States

Between 1975 and 1982, the annual number of women who died for reasons related to reproduction declined from 1,083 to 751. . . . This decline continues the trend noted since 1955, with a slight decrease in the rate of that decline. . . . In 1982, the overall adjusted reproductive mortality rate was 2.2 deaths per 100,000 women at risk, a 35 per cent decrease since 1975. Each component of the adjusted reproductive mortality rate also decreased: maternal mortality dropped by 35 per cent, abortion mortality by 89 per cent, and contraceptive mortality by 35 per cent . . . . By 1982, the mortality rate for induced (legalized) abortion had dropped to nearly zero, making it a minor component of reproductive mortality.

From *AJPH*, July 1987, pp. 834–835

52 YEARS AGO

Legal Abortion and Public Health

Legalization of induced abortion has been followed by a decline in abortion deaths, a decrease in the hospitalization of women with the complications of abortion, lower out-of-wedlock birth rates, and improved infant health. As recently as 1930, abortion was the certified cause of death for almost 2,700 American women in a single year. . . . In 1971, the first full calendar year

AJPH March 2026, Vol. 116, No. 3

State-level abortion restrictions have been linked to worsening maternal and infant health outcomes. Some states with bans have recently reported substantial increases in maternal mortality, sepsis in pregnancy, congenital anomalies, and infant deaths, disproportionately affecting marginalized populations and widening existing inequities.[8] Yet, the post-*Dobbs* data regarding state-level abortion bans on maternal and infant outcomes are very limited.

Post-*Dobbs* restrictions and cutbacks also strain the health care workforce and public health data infrastructure. Training in abortion care has been severely curtailed, particularly in states with bans, exacerbating shortages in trained gynecologists and obstetricians and expanding "maternity care deserts," especially in underserved areas.[9] Current ongoing federal reductions in workforce and funding for reproductive and maternal health data systems hinder efforts to monitor the impact of restrictive abortion policies. Strengthening public health data infrastructure and monitoring systems is vital for understanding and addressing the consequences of restrictive abortion policies.

Since the *AJPH* October 2024 issue featuring abortion access two years after the *Dobbs* decision,[10] the *Journal* has remained committed to spotlighting this public health topic through evidence-based research and balanced opinions. The following summarizes the articles in this special section, covering the reframing of reproductive autonomy possibly as violence, importance of maternal health data transparency, impacts of states' bans on abortions and maternal and infant health, and effects of states' bans on neighboring protective states that serve as destinations for abortion care seekers. Our intent is to present rigorous scientific inquiry and innovative thinking as abortion policies continue to evolve.

REFRAMING REPRODUCTIVE AUTONOMY

Reproductive autonomy is the right of individuals to make informed, self-guided decisions about their reproductive health. Santaularia Gomez et al. (p. 329) argue that policies limiting reproductive autonomy constitute acts of violence. They present three examples—limits on sex education, abortion, and parental leave—as ways that the government leverages its power to support and constrain reproductive autonomy across the life course. They define these limits as critical human rights issues with far-reaching harms. Yamin (p. 321) agrees that restricting reproductive autonomy could be framed as violence, consistent with concepts of freedom from obstetric violence. However, the author questions the intentionality of legislators to oppress women and the effectiveness of criminalization as a remedy compared with education and regulation.

MATERNAL HEALTH DATA TRANSPARENCY AND REPORTING

The United States has the highest maternal mortality rate of any high-income country,[11] and evidence now links restricted abortion access to this increase. Fletcher et al. (p. 323) used the Texas Maternal Mortality and Morbidity Review Committee as a case example. The Committee's recent decision to withhold maternal health data for the first two years after the state's abortion ban offers a

Continued on page 319...

HISTORY CORNER

following the passage of New York State's legalized abortion law, and the first year in which the number of nationally reported abortions neared 500,000, only 99 women in the United States died from causes related to abortion. Data collected through a special inquiry of state and selected city health departments in 1972 and 1973 indicate that this decline is continuing. . . .

Certainly the legalization of abortion has not been without problems. When the legal restrictions were first removed from the practice of abortion, few physicians had formal training in performing this operation. As abortion became legalized on a state-by-state basis, the interstate travel of women seeking legal abortion disrupted the continuity of care which a pregnant woman customarily received in this country and preventable death and disease were associated with this disruption.

From *AJPH*, August 1974, p. 823–824

55 YEARS AGO

Recommended Standards for Abortion Services

Since 1967, 15 states have responded to the increasing public demand for changes in the legal restriction of abortion practice by passing new laws. Moreover, at least 14 states have had the constitutionality of their abortion laws challenged in court. Public health agencies must be prepared, therefore, to respond to an increasing need for abortion services.

preview of post–*Dobbs*-era data reporting approaches. This editorial stresses that transparent maternal health data, monitoring, and reporting are crucial for evidence-based decision-making, accountability, health equity, and building public trust.

ABORTIONS IN STATES WITH BANS

While previous studies document a decrease in overall abortions in states with bans, they have not detailed age-specific postban changes. In 2021, Texas banned abortion upon detection of embryonic cardiac activity (around five to six weeks after the last menstrual period). White et al. (p. 337) found this law disproportionately affected facility-based abortion access care for individuals aged 24 years and younger. This ban compounded existing barriers for minors and young adults, including parental involvement laws and other obstacles to facility-based care.

MATERNAL AND INFANT HEALTH IN STATES WITH BANS

Severe maternal morbidity includes unexpected outcomes of labor and delivery that can result in substantial short-term and long-term health consequences. Siegal and Soni (p. 341) add to this literature by examining how state laws imposing gestational limits on abortion impact severe maternal morbidity hospitalization rates nationwide, using a difference-in-differences approach with longitudinal state-level data. They find that states with these restrictions have significantly higher severe maternal morbidity hospitalization rates, which disproportionately affect older patients, those with public insurance, and individuals from low-income communities.

Until now, no post-*Dobbs* evidence-based research has examined the effect of the new state abortion restrictions on birth outcomes beyond preliminary infant mortality data.[12] Using the first 18 months of post-*Dobbs* birth data, Wallace et al. (p. 345) found that the monthly birth rates and preterm births among non-Hispanic Black women in the states with abortion bans increased by 3.5% and 2.1%, respectively, compared with expected levels absent a ban.

ABORTIONS IN NEIGHBORING STATES WITHOUT BANS

As the patchwork of restrictions shifts, new research examines how state bans impact abortion access in neighboring states that protect abortion access. Smith et al. (p. 351) examined data from three health clinics in Michigan—where abortion remains legal with no gestational limit—near borders with Ohio (ban 2022–2023) and Indiana (ban 2023–present). They found significant increases in clinic visits, patients undergoing later-gestation abortions, and use of medication abortions compared with the previous year's data.

Similarly, Illinois has emerged as an abortion care haven because of strong patient and provider protections. Using granular data comparing monthly changes 12 months before and after *Dobbs*, Smith et al. (p. 359) found a 35% increase in facility-based abortions, driven by a 191% increase in out-of-state patients. They observed a 53% increase in facility-based abortions, 22% increase in medication abortions, and 75% increase in abortion at 12 weeks gestation and later.

Continued on page 320...

HISTORY CORNER

Abortion services are an integral part of comprehensive family planning and maternal and child health care. As such, abortion and contraceptive counseling and services should be available together Contraception should be encouraged as a means of minimizing the need for abortion. Counseling and services for abortion and contraception should receive full administrative and financial support as part of maternal and child health programs.

From *AJPH*, February 1971, p. 396.

These findings from Michigan and Illinois provide emerging evidence that protective states neighboring those with restrictive state laws act as destinations for those seeking abortion care. Redd et al. (p. 326) writes that, in this environment, abortion-protective states have the opportunity to implement policies to expand access, support clinics handling the influx of out-of-state patients, and protect the abortion care workforce. AJPH

ABOUT THE AUTHORS

Denys T. Lau is the *AJPH* Editor-in-Chief and is with the Johns Hopkins University, Baltimore, MD; George Washington University, Washington, DC; and University of Illinois at Chicago. Jihong Liu is an *AJPH* Associate Editor and is with the Department of Epidemiology and Biostatistics, University of South Carolina, Columbia. Marian Moser Jones is an *AJPH* Associate Editor and is with the College of Public Health, The Ohio State University, Columbus.

CORRESPONDENCE

Correspondence should be sent to Denys T. Lau, Editor-in-Chief, *American Journal of Public Health*, 800 I St NW, Washington, DC 20001 (e-mail: denys.lau@apha.org). Reprints can be ordered at https://www.ajph.org by clicking the "Reprints" link.

PUBLICATION INFORMATION

Full Citation: Lau DT, Liu J, Jones MM. Post-*Dobbs* era: evolving abortion care restrictions and public health impact. *Am J Public Health*. 2026;116(3):317–320.

Acceptance Date: December 16, 2025.

DOI: https://doi.org/10.2105/AJPH.2025.308394

CONTRIBUTORS

D. T. Lau drafted the editorial. M. M. Jones and J. Liu revised the text. D. T. Lau and M. M. Jones participated in the editorial processes for the special section.

CONFLICTS OF INTEREST

The authors declare no conflicts.

REFERENCES

1. Kaiser Family Foundation. Abortion in the United States Dashboard. Available at: https://www.kff.org/womens-health-policy/abortion-in-the-u-s-dashboard. Accessed December 15, 2025.
2. Egervary C. How the US abortion landscape stacks up to international recommendations. *Fordham International Law Journal Online*. April 2, 2024. Available at: https://www.fordhamilj.org/iljonline/how-the-us-abortion-landscape-stacks-up-to-international-recommendations. Accessed December 15, 2025.
3. Center for Reproductive Rights. Interstate shield laws. June 26, 2024. Available at: https://reproductiverights.org/resources/interstate-shield-laws. Accessed December 15, 2025.
4. Kimport K, Schroeder R, Rocca CH. Caller volume and gestational length at an abortion fund after *Dobbs*. *JAMA Netw Open*. 2025;8(12):e2546508. https://doi.org/10.1001/jamanetworkopen.2025.46508
5. Woskie LR, Brower N, Shaffer J, Ladin K. Obstetric-related emergency medical treatment and Labor Act violations and no health exception bans. *JAMA Health Forum*. 2025;6(12):e254726. https://doi.org/10.1001/jamahealthforum.2025.4726
6. Aiken ARA, Scott JG, Gomperts R. Provision of abortion medications using online asynchronous telemedicine under shield laws in the US. *JAMA*. 2025 21;334(15):1388–1390. https://doi.org/10.1001/jama.2025.11420
7. Addante AN, Eisenberg DL, Valentine MC, Leonard J, Joynt Maddox DE, Hoofnagle MH. The association between state-level abortion restrictions and maternal mortality in the United States, 1995–2017. *Contraception*. 2021;104(5):496–501. https://doi.org/10.1016/j.contraception.2021.03.018
8. Cwiak C. The far-reaching health implications of the *Dobbs* decision. *JAMA Netw Open*. 2025;8(12):e2546416. https://doi.org/10.1001/jamanetworkopen.2025.46416
9. Frederiksen B, Ranji U, Gomez I, Salganicof A. A national survey of OBGYNs' experiences after *Dobbs*. Kaiser Family Foundation. June 21, 2023. Available at: https://www.kff.org/womens-health-policy/a-national-survey-of-obgyns-experiences-after-dobbs. Accessed December 15, 2025.
10. Kapadia F, Ferguson L, Parmet WE. Understanding the post-*Dobbs* landscape for abortion care in the United States. *Am J Public Health*. 2024;114(10):994–996. https://doi.org/10.2105/AJPH.2024.307827
11. Gunja MZ, Gumas ED, Masitha R, Zephyrin LC. Insights into the US maternal mortality crisis: an international comparison. Issue Brief. The Commonwealth Fund. June 4, 2024. Available at: https://www.commonwealthfund.org/publications/issue-briefs/2024/jun/insights-us-maternal-mortality-crisis-international-comparison. Accessed December 15, 2025.
12. Gemmill A, Franks AM, Anjur-Dietrich S, et al. US abortion bans and infant mortality. *JAMA*. 2025;333(15):1315–1323. https://doi.org/10.1001/jama.2024.28517

Structural Violence and Reproductive Justice

Alicia Ely Yamin, JD, PhD, MPH

ABOUT THE AUTHOR

Alicia Ely Yamin is a lecturer on law at Harvard Law School, Cambridge, MA, and adjunct senior lecturer on health policy and management, Harvard T. H. Chan School of Public Health, Boston, MA.

See also Abortion and Public Health Impact in Post-*Dobbs* Era, pp. 321–367.

In this issue of *AJPH,* Santaularia Gomez et al. (p. 329) argue that policies and laws that restrict reproductive autonomy constitute forms of violence, highlighting three examples: sex education, abortion restrictions, and parental leave policies. In framing restrictions on reproductive autonomy as violence, the authors take up arguments that have been well-developed in the context of obstetric care. The concept of obstetric violence emerged out of feminists' struggle for humanized deliveries (*partos humanizados*) in Latin America in the 1970s but has spread far beyond the region and has been widely adopted in both domestic constitutional and international law.[1]

The authors cite the definition of violence from the World Health Organization (WHO) as the basis for their organizing framework:

> the intentional use of physical force or power, threatened or actual, against oneself, another person, or against a group or community, that either results in or has a high likelihood of resulting in injury, death, psychological harm, maldevelopment or deprivation (p. 330).

Although Santaularia Gomez et al. argue that the inclusion of power greatly expands the scope of what we consider violence, in practice, the WHO has eschewed the broader concept of "obstetric violence" to focus on the much narrower "disrespect and abuse."

OBSTETRIC VIOLENCE

The concept of "obstetric violence"—as opposed to "disrespect and abuse"—challenges the paradigm of medicalized maternal health care in which the physician is the protagonist of the process and exercises power over the pregnant person's body, while her knowledge and feelings are treated as irrelevant to the technical task of delivery.[2] The denial of agency involved in obstetric violence is enacted by individual providers but often stems from broader structural forces, such as austerity policies that constrain the provision of services.[3] Thus, obstetric violence—and arguably the other issues cited by the authors—constitute particular examples of the late Paul Farmer's framing of structural violence, defined as

> *structural* because they are embedded in the political and economic organization of our social world [and] *violent* because they cause injury to people [emphasis added].[4(p1686)]

GENDER-BASED VIOLENCE

More broadly, conceptualizing freedom from violence in human rights terms has been key to denaturalizing the treatment of women in domestic spaces as well as health systems. In the 1990s, Rhonda Copelon argued that domestic violence—historically excluded from human rights protections because it was not perpetrated directly by state agents—met the criteria for "cruel, inhuman and degrading treatment" under international law.[5] Feminists argued that the inaction of the state in failing to prevent, sanction, and eradicate domestic violence was a political—and legal—choice.[6] In 1999, the South African Constitutional Court suggested it was essential to shift our understanding of the suffering produced by widespread domestic violence from a "misfortune to be endured into injustice to be remedied."[7] Subsequently, domestic and intimate partner violence have been read into legal frameworks prohibiting torture and cruel, inhuman, and degrading treatment, including naming them as violations of peremptory norms under international law.[8]

Likewise, the arguments of Santaularia Gomez et al. regarding abortion restrictions after *Dobbs* find resonance in the successful efforts by feminist movements to reframe draconian restrictions on abortion in terms of pervasive gender-based violence in domestic constitutional law.[9] These arguments have been taken up in international law as well, including in a General Comment from the Committee on the Elimination of Discrimination Against Women.[8] Although the United States has not ratified the relevant treaties under international law, drawing on these

AJPH March 2026, Vol. 116, No. 3

conceptualizations regarding freedom from violence in obstetric care as well as abortion is growing in both legal and other advocacy.[10]

LEGAL DEFINITIONS AND IMPLICATIONS

Although I agree with the authors' aims, labeling the passage of such varied legislation as violence raises complicated questions regarding what harms count under the law. That is, the aim as well as likely impact of legislation may be contested; for some of us, banning sex work is deploying the police powers of the state to commit violence and oppression against women and sexual minorities; for others, the failure to pass such legislation might constitute violence against women.

Second, if the reframing as violence is a "call to action," as the authors argue, the remedy for such "violent acts" would likely be found in criminal law. Where that has occurred in the context of obstetric violence, it has been enormously controversial, as doing so not only reinserts reproductive activity into criminal law, from which advocates have long sought to remove it, but also sets up a potential conflict between physicians and patients that can lead to less availability of quality care.[11] In the context of growing maternity care deserts in the United States, the patients who are most likely to suffer unintended consequences are impoverished and disproportionately Brown and Black pregnant persons with the fewest options.

Third, what about all the other legislation, which is broader and often economic in nature, such as the impending drastic reductions in Medicaid spending per President Trump's One Big Beautiful Bill Act, which will foreseeably cause restrictions on reproductive health and autonomy?

Indeed, so much of sexual and reproductive health and justice lies in contested domains at the intersection of private morality and public policy, and between political questions and judicially enforceable rights, raises complicated issues. Nonetheless, hard-won lessons from reproductive justice movements across the world have shown that it is critical to deploy innovative framings to denaturalize abuse that is taken for granted, and in the United States, we should learn from those efforts. Understanding how structural violence in political economy factors as well as gender and health policies impact sexual and reproductive health must be part of that struggle. AJPH

CORRESPONDENCE

Correspondence should be sent to Alicia Ely Yamin, Harvard Law School, 23 Everett St, Room 322, Cambridge, MA 02138 (e-mail: ayamin@law.harvard.edu). Reprints can be ordered at https://www.ajph.org by clicking the "Reprints" link.

PUBLICATION INFORMATION

Full Citation: Yamin AE. Structural violence and reproductive justice. *Am J Public Health*. 2026; 116(3):321–322.

Acceptance Date: November 9, 2025.

DOI: https://doi.org/10.2105/AJPH.2025.308357

CONFLICTS OF INTEREST

The author declares no conflicts of interest.

REFERENCES

1. Pickles C. "Everything is obstetric violence now": identifying the violence in "obstetric violence" to strengthen socio-legal reform efforts. *Oxf J Leg Stud*. 2024;44(3):616–644. https://doi.org/10.1093/ojls/gqae016
2. United Nations General Assembly. A human rights-based approach to mistreatment and violence against women in reproductive health services with a focus on childbirth and obstetric violence. Document no. A/74/137. July 11, 2019. Available at: https://docs.un.org/en/A/74/137. Accessed November 30, 2025.
3. Human Rights Watch. No Money for Care: Obstetric Violence in Sierra Leone. 2025. Available at: https://www.hrw.org/report/2025/11/02/no-money-no-care/obstetric-violence-in-sierra-leone. Accessed November 30, 2025.
4. Farmer PE, Nizeye B, Stulac S, Keshavjee S. Structural violence and clinical medicine. *PLoS Med*. 2006;3(10):e449. https://doi.org/10.1371/journal.pmed.0030449
5. Copelon R. Intimate terror: understanding domestic violence as torture. In: Cook RJ, ed. *Human Rights of Women: National and International Perspectives*. Philadelphia, PA: University of Pennsylvania Press; 2012:116–152.
6. Sifris R. *Reproductive Freedom, Torture and International Human Rights: Challenging the Masculinisation of Torture*. 1st ed. London, England: Routledge; 2014.
7. *S v Baloyi* et al. (J. Albie Sachs) CCT (South Africa) 00 29/99 1999, para 12.
8. Convention on the Elimination of All Forms of Discrimination Against Women. General recommendation No. 35 on gender-based violence against women, updating general recommendation No. 19. Document no. CEDAW/C/GC/35. July 26, 2017. Available at: https://docs.un.org/en/CEDAW/C/GC/35. Accessed November 30, 2025.
9. Corte Constitucional de Colombia. C-555/2022. 2022. Available at: https://www.corteconstitucional.gov.co/relatoria/2022/c-055-22.htm. Accessed December 2, 2025.
10. Vullikanti M, Yamin AE. Contesting power abuses and pregnancy paradigms: understanding obstetric violence as structural violence. In: Moore A, Price J, eds. *Handbook of Structural Violence*. Berlin, Germany: DeGruyter; 2026. In press.
11. Chervenak F, McLeod-Sordjan R, Pollet S, et al. Obstetric violence is a misnomer. *Am J Obstet Gynecol*. 2024;230(3S):S1138–S1145. https://doi.org/10.1016/j.ajog.2023.10.003

Post-*Dobbs* Realities: Ethical Imperatives for Data Transparency and Trust in Maternal Health Care

Faith E. Fletcher, PhD, MA, Sophie L. Schott, BA, Kelley Akhiemokhali, MA, and Kari White, PhD, MPH

ABOUT THE AUTHORS

Faith E. Fletcher and Kelley Akhiemokhali are with the Center for Medical Ethics and Health Policy, Baylor College of Medicine, Houston, TX. Sophie L. Schott is with McGovern Medical School, UTHealth Houston, Houston, TX. Kari White is with Resound Research for Reproductive Health and the Baker Institute for Public Policy, Rice University, Houston, TX.

See also Abortion and Public Health Impact in Post-*Dobbs* Era, pp. 321–367.

Following the US Supreme Court's decision in *Dobbs v Jackson Women's Health Org.* (No. 19-1392, slip op. at 5 [US June 24, 2022]), which unraveled the federal constitutional right to abortion, officials in Georgia, Idaho, Arkansas, and Texas took steps to modify, limit, or dismantle their maternal mortality review committees (MMRCs).[1] State MMRCs are uniquely positioned to evaluate maternal health outcomes, including the effects of abortion bans, and to offer evidence-based guidance to prevent future pregnancy-related morbidity and mortality. MMRCs also contribute to national efforts to monitor maternal health trends through standardized data reports to the Centers for Disease Control and Prevention's (CDC) Maternal Mortality Review Information Application System.[2] By limiting MMRCs' activities, states disregard the public health consequences of abortion bans and undermine efforts to advance maternal health equity. These actions further contribute to the public's lack of confidence in essential public health systems.

Recent actions by the Texas Maternal Mortality and Morbidity Review Committee (MMMRC) offer a preview of how other states might restrict or delay maternal health data reporting in the post-*Dobbs* era and underscore the urgent need for data transparency to advance health equity.[1] Importantly, Texas is a key driver of national maternal health policy: It has the second highest number of births—more than 10% of all births in the United States—and its maternal death rate far exceeds the national average.[3] Texas implemented its abortion ban a year before the *Dobbs* decision through the passage of Texas Senate Bill 8, also known as the Texas Heartbeat Act, which prohibits abortion after the detection of fetal cardiac activity, typically around six weeks of gestation.[4] In addition to being the most populous state to have enacted an abortion ban, Texas is currently the only state not participating in the CDC's Maternal Mortality Review Information Application System, thus limiting the state's ability to contribute to and benefit from standardized maternal health data and insights shared across states.[2] As a result, Texas is considered a key case study in understanding the early impacts of restrictive abortion legislation.

Before the *Dobbs* decision, experts warned against delaying the release of public health data, emphasizing that such delays interfered with efforts to reduce preventable maternal deaths. However, on September 2, 2022—just one day after the Texas MMMRC report was due—the Texas Department of State Health Services commissioner, who oversees the MMMRC, announced that there would be at least a nine-month delay in the release of the report (Figure 1). The commissioner defended the decision and stated that the delay was to ensure that all cohort deaths were included in the report. Following sustained pressure from public health professionals, advocates, and maternal health experts (including an open letter from the Society for Maternal–Fetal Medicine[5]), the MMMRC eventually released the report in December 2022.

In March 2024, around the time when the next Texas MMMRC biennial report was scheduled for release, committee members learned that they were not permitted to scrutinize abortion ban–related deaths. Maternal deaths linked to delays and denials of care owing to abortion bans should fall under the purview of MMRCs, but since the inception of the MMMRC in 2013, the committee has never been allowed to review such cases. This directive is alarming and will result in undercounting pregnancy-related deaths.[6] In September 2024, the Texas MMMRC announced that maternal deaths occurring in 2022 and 2023 would not be

AJPH March 2026, Vol. 116, No. 3

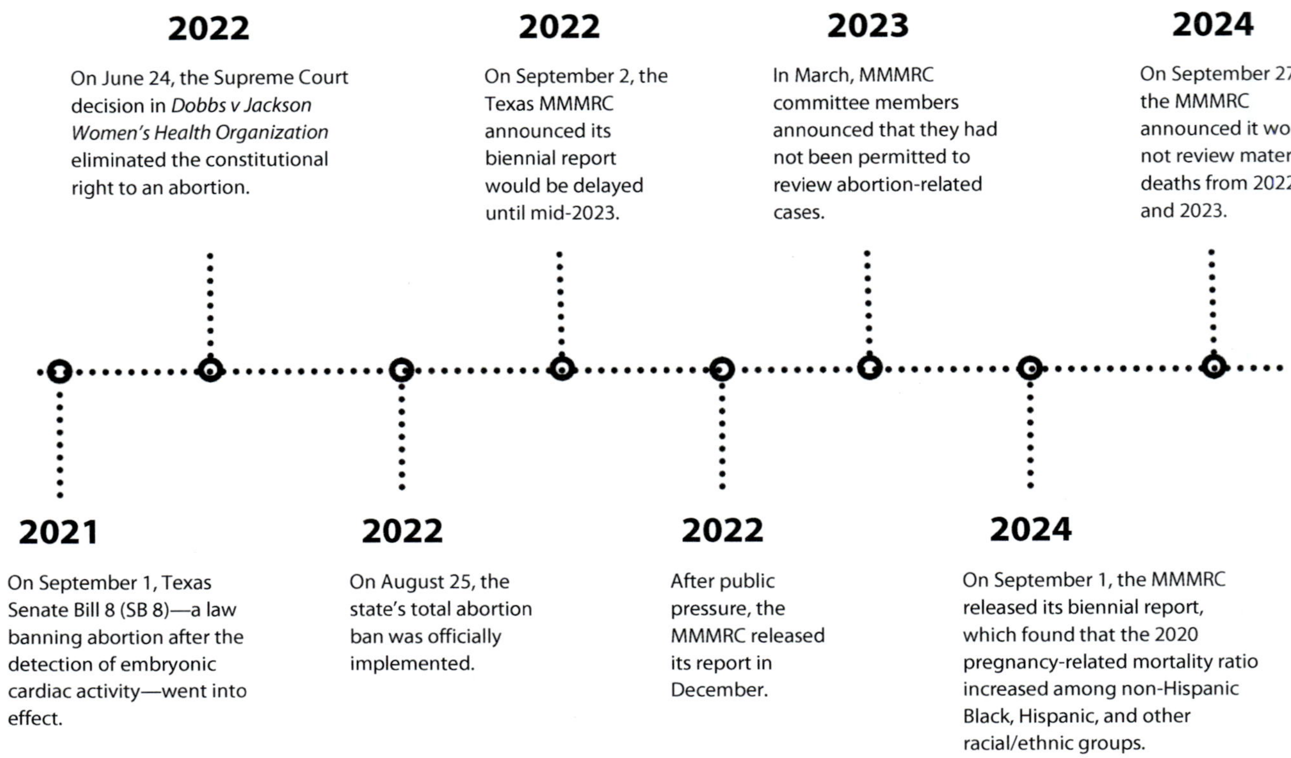

FIGURE 1— Post-*Dobbs* Data Transparency: Key Maternal Events, Texas, 2021–2024

MMMRC = Maternal Mortality and Morbidity Review Committee

analyzed. The committee's chair argued that foregoing analysis of 2022 and 2023 data was not concerning, as future cohorts would be subject to the same legal landscape. This argument was misguided. Simply put, the failure to analyze these data limits the MMMRC's ability to understand the real-time impacts of abortion bans on maternal and child health in Texas. Importantly, researchers have projected that abortion bans could lead to a 21% increase in overall US maternal mortality and a 33% increase in pregnancy-related deaths among Black Americans.[7] These stark estimates reflect existing inequities: Black women in the United States are two to three times more likely to die during childbirth than are their White counterparts. Thus, the failure to release current maternal data—intended to evaluate disparities and guide public health decisions—raises concerns about the trustworthiness of systems charged with protecting public health.

Public health ethics guidelines emphasize that data transparency requires open communication, stakeholder engagement, and a willingness to share information—even when unfavorable—to promote public trust and accountability for public health actions and decisions.[8] Ethical and timely dissemination of data, particularly in maternal and child health, has not only revolutionized public health practices but also shaped medical guidelines, clinical interventions, and policy decision-making. In the absence of timely and transparent data, affected populations are made invisible in policy and public health decision-making processes, undermining efforts to advance equitable resource allocation, effective program design, and responsive clinical practices.[9] Notably, as reported recently in *The Dallas Morning News*, two Texas mothers in need of abortion-related procedures died after being denied timely medical care following pregnancy complications. These deaths underscore the need to evaluate and document the real-world impact of abortion bans, particularly on reproductive health care, rights, and justice.[10]

By refusing to comprehensively review maternal deaths, the Texas MMMRC is deviating from established public health best practices and obscuring the deadly consequences of restricted access to essential reproductive health care. The MMMRC's ability to provide actionable recommendations is weakened when the available data are incomplete or flawed. These actions occur against a backdrop of ongoing cuts to federal public health programs and the suspension of long-standing population-based maternal health surveillance efforts, such as the Pregnancy Risk Assessment Monitoring System. Furthermore, suppressing essential public health data compromises public trust, which arguably may be one of the most valuable assets in public health.[8] The erosion of trust and transparency is especially troubling given the broader national crisis in maternal and infant health. For example, the Mississippi State Department of Health recently declared a public health emergency in response to rising infant mortality rates across the state.[11] To effectively address these disparities nationwide, efforts must prioritize maternal health through high-quality prenatal and postpartum care, expanded access to mental health and social resources, and the implementation of more robust data collection methods. Public health evidence must guide efforts to meet community needs long before a crisis unfolds.[12]

The success of public health policies, practices, and actions relies heavily on gaining public trust. As key informants of public health policy, state MMRCs in Texas and beyond have an ethical responsibility to release data on present-day maternal deaths—which are avoidable, preventable, and unjust—in a timely and transparent manner. To be clear, suppressing and withholding data not only hinders public health and clinical action but also undermines ongoing efforts to build institutional trustworthiness,[13] an essential priority in today's public health and medical landscape.[14] As health professionals, we must not allow the delayed release or suppression of critical public health data to become normalized. This moment calls for prioritizing justice as a core principle of public health and demands a critical examination and dismantling of harmful practices embedded in systems, sectors, and institutions.[15] AJPH

CORRESPONDENCE

Correspondence should be sent to Faith E. Fletcher, 1 Baylor Plaza, Suite 310DK, Houston, TX 77030 (e-mail: Faith.Fletcher@bcm.edu). Reprints can be ordered at https://www.ajph.org by clicking the "Reprints" link.

PUBLICATION INFORMATION

Full Citation: Fletcher FE, Schott SL, Akhiemokhali K, White K. Post-*Dobbs* realities: ethical imperatives for data transparency and trust in maternal health care. *Am J Public Health*. 2026;116(3):323–325.

Acceptance Date: October 14, 2025.

DOI: https://doi.org/10.2105/AJPH.2025.308343

ORCID iDs:

Faith E. Fletcher https://orcid.org/0000-0001-8075-6112

Sophie L. Schott https://orcid.org/0000-0003-3003-3420

Kelley Akhiemokhali https://orcid.org/0009-0009-4535-1211

CONTRIBUTORS

The authors contributed equally to the development and writing of this editorial.

ACKNOWLEDGMENTS

This work was supported by the Greenwall Faculty Scholars Program in Bioethics (grant to F. E. Fletcher).

Special thanks to I. Glenn Cohen, JD, for providing valuable early feedback.

Note. Any opinions, conclusions, and recommendations expressed in this editorial are those of the authors and do not represent the views of Baylor College of Medicine, UTHealth Houston, or Rice University.

CONFLICTS OF INTEREST

The authors have no conflicts of interest to disclose.

REFERENCES

1. Klibanoff E. Texas' maternal mortality committee faces backlash for not reviewing deaths from first two years post-*Dobbs*. *The Texas Tribune*. December 6, 2024. Available at: https://www.texastribune.org/2024/12/06/texas-maternal-mortality-committee-deaths. Accessed February 17, 2025.
2. Centers for Disease Control and Prevention. Enhancing reviews and surveillance to eliminate maternal mortality. Maternal mortality prevention. August 7, 2024. Available at: https://www.cdc.gov/maternal-mortality/php/erase-mm/index.html. Accessed August 11, 2025.
3. Arey W, Lerma K, Beasley A, Harper L, Moayedi G, White K. A preview of the dangerous future of abortion bans—Texas Senate Bill 8. *N Engl J Med*. 2022;387(5):388–390. https://doi.org/10.1056/NEJMp2207423
4. Lampe JR, Shimabukuro JO. The Texas Heartbeat Act (S.B. 8), *Whole Woman's Health v. Jackson, and United States v. Texas*: frequently asked questions. Available at: https://www.congress.gov/crs-product/LSB10651. Accessed October 1, 2025.
5. Society for Maternal-Fetal Medicine. Demand for compliance with Section 34.015 of the Texas Health & Safety Code. November 2, 2022. Available at: https://democracyforward.org/wp-content/uploads/2022/11/SMFM-Demand-Letter-DSHS-MMMRC-11.2.22.pdf. Accessed August 11, 2025.
6. Centers for Disease Control and Prevention. Abortion surveillance—United States, 2022. *MMWR Surveill Summ*. 2024;73(7):1–28. https://doi.org/10.15585/mmwr.ss7307a1
7. Stevenson AJ. One component of the mortality impact of a total US abortion ban: a research note on the mortality consequence of denying all wanted induced abortions. *Demography*. 2021;58(6):2019–2028. https://doi.org/10.1215/00703370-9585908
8. American Public Health Association. Public health code of ethics. Available at: https://www.apha.org/getcontentasset/43d5fdee-4ccd-427d-90db-b1d585c880b0/7ca0dc9d-611d-46e2-9fd3-26a4c03ddcbb/code_of_ethics.pdf. Accessed October 1, 2025.
9. Braveman P, Arkin E, Kauh T, Holm N. Health equity: everyone counts. May 1, 2022. Available at: https://www.rwjf.org/en/insights/our-research/2022/05/health-equity–everyone-counts.html. Accessed August 1, 2025.
10. Rice WS, Hartwig SA, McMahon HV, et al. Collective persistence, care, and advocacy amid repeated attacks on reproductive freedom. *Am J Public Health*. 2024;114(10):1000–1002. https://doi.org/10.2105/AJPH.2024.307810
11. Mississippi State Department of Health. MSDH declares public health emergency on infant mortality. August 21, 2025. Available at: https://msdh.ms.gov/page/23,30305,341.html. Accessed September 26, 2025.
12. Akhiemokhali K, Fletcher FE. Midwives are essential for improving Mississippi's maternal and infant health. Available at: https://www.thehastingscenter.org/midwives-are-essential-for-improving-mississippis-maternal-and-infant-health. Accessed October 27, 2025.
13. Best AL, Fletcher FE, Kadono M, Warren RC. Institutional distrust among African Americans and building trustworthiness in the COVID-19 response: implications for ethical public health practice. *J Health Care Poor Underserved*. 2021;32(1):90–98. https://doi.org/10.1353/hpu.2021.0010
14. Muigai W. Trusted messengers: public health education and advocacy in 20th century Black American newspapers. *Am J Public Health*. 2025;115(3):326–332. https://doi.org/10.2105/AJPH.2024.307897
15. Fletcher FE, Jiang W, Best AL. Antiracist praxis in public health: a call for ethical reflections. *Hastings Cent Rep*. 2021;51(2):6–9. https://doi.org/10.1002/hast.1240

The Opportunity of Abortion-Protective States in the Post-*Dobbs* Era: Implications for Public Health Policy and Practice

Sara K. Redd, PhD, MSPH, Sofia Filippa, MPH, Alina A. Luke, MPH, Hayley V. McMahon, MSPH, and Emma Chew Murphy, MD

ABOUT THE AUTHORS

Sara K. Redd, Sofia Filippa, Alina A. Luke, and Hayley V. McMahon are with the Center for Reproductive Health Research in the Southeast (RISE) and the Department of Behavioral, Social, and Health Education Sciences, Rollins School of Public Health, Emory University, Atlanta, GA. Emma Chew Murphy is with the Department of Obstetrics, Gynecology, and Reproductive Sciences, University of California, San Francisco.

See also Abortion and Public Health Impact in Post-*Dobbs* Era, pp. 321–367.

The June 2022 US Supreme Court's decision in *Dobbs v Jackson Women's Health Organization* (*Dobbs*) fundamentally restructured the US abortion care landscape. In this post-*Dobbs* environment, abortion-protective states like Illinois, as explored by Smith et al. in this issue of *AJPH* (p. 359), play an increasingly critical role in an actively evolving abortion care ecosystem. Their analysis of data from two large Illinois abortion providers highlights the collective impact of Illinois's efforts to expand access to abortion—through state-, community-, and clinic-level policies and practices—on in- and out-of-state patients' ability to access abortion after *Dobbs*. These findings have critical public health policy and practice implications, demonstrating the opportunity for states to implement policies at multiple levels to expand access to care and serve as critical access points amid an increasingly hostile political and legal environment. Furthermore, the findings of Smith et al. emphasize the importance of protecting the well-being of the abortion care workforce given growing demands[1] and persistent and increasing violence from antiabortion groups.[2]

PUBLIC HEALTH POLICY IMPLICATIONS

Smith et al. analyzed data before and after *Dobbs* from two Illinois-based clinics that implemented numerous policies expanding access to care: offering procedural abortion at medication abortion–only sites, delivering medication abortion via telemedicine, and expanding gestational limits. Their findings show a 35% increase in patient volume after *Dobbs*, suggesting that these policies supported access for a larger patient pool. Growing evidence supports the efficacy and safety of medication abortion via telehealth, which offers expanded access for individuals in rural areas or with logistical or transportation barriers to in-clinic appointments. Amid the pervasive presence of antiabortion protestors, abortion stigma, and potential concerns about legal restrictions, abortion patients may prefer the privacy and confidentiality afforded by telemedicine.

Notably, clinic-based abortion care in or beyond the second trimester has historically been limited, more so after *Dobbs*. Between 2021 and 2023, 20% of facilities nationwide decreased their gestational limits, and the number of facilities offering care at or after 24 weeks decreased by 16.7%.[3] Laws banning or restricting abortion by gestation delay care, resulting in more patients seeking abortion later in pregnancy.[4] Abortions at or beyond 12 weeks increased by 75% after *Dobbs* at clinics analyzed by Smith et al., underscoring how increased gestational limits expand access to care and Illinois's status as a receiving state. As the authors highlight, combining clinic-led change to expand abortion at later gestations with community-level efforts to invest in patient support resources, including patient navigation and partnership with local abortion funds, are particularly crucial in a post-*Dobbs* context.

Illinois has established itself as a hub for abortion access, largely through implementing multiple state-level policies reducing barriers to and increasing structural support for abortion care. As outlined by Smith et al., these policies include requiring Medicaid and private health insurance to cover abortion, establishing a right to make individual decisions about reproductive health (including abortion), repealing a parental notification law, and enacting a shield law protecting out-of-state patients receiving care in Illinois and Illinois providers from out-of-state surveillance and prosecution. Furthermore, Illinois expanded the scope of practice to allow advanced practice clinicians to provide abortions, allocated state funding for abortion care, and changed state data collection and reporting practices to protect patient privacy. The findings of Smith et al.—including a 191% increase in out-of-state patients while maintaining in-state volume—demonstrate how these policies have created a protective environment that has reduced barriers for abortion seekers and enabled the health care system to expand its capacity to support the influx of patients from other states.

PUBLIC HEALTH PRACTICE IMPLICATIONS

In the study by Smith et al., out-of-state patients increased from roughly 4500 before *Dobbs* to more than 13 000 after *Dobbs*. While most came from neighboring Midwestern states, the largest percentage increases came from Southern states (e.g., Alabama, Florida, Louisiana) and Arizona. These findings align with those from the Guttmacher Institute's Monthly Abortion Provision Study, which suggests that more than 39 000 people from 16 states in the Midwest and South traveled to Illinois for abortion care in 2023.[5] Traveling out of state for care represents a significant burden—requiring an immense amount of logistical, financial, and emotional resources—particularly for those traveling hundreds or even thousands of miles. The study reveals notable increases in people traveling long distances after *Dobbs*, from as far as Arizona, Florida, and Texas, demonstrating Illinois's position as a major care hub for people in abortion deserts across the country. Notably, states and municipalities in protective environments like Illinois and California have allocated funds to offset costs for individuals traveling long distance for abortion care.

Supporting Clinics in Abortion-Protective Settings

Given the crucial role that Illinois and other abortion-protective states play in facilitating abortion access for people nationwide, it is increasingly imperative to provide support for clinics striving to meet the influx of need. Clinics in restrictive and supportive states alike have struggled to stay open, working to make abortion financially accessible while balancing the costs of extensive security measures, facility maintenance, equipment and supplies, and adequate staffing.[6] In states ensuring Medicaid coverage for abortion, clinics continue to face the challenge of low Medicaid reimbursement rates for services.[7] Illinois has emerged as a model in this respect, aligning Medicaid reimbursement rates with out-of-pocket charges,[7] thereby providing greater stability to clinics. As many clinics face challenges with provider retention,[8] there remains a pressing need for states to follow Illinois's lead by investing in abortion education for clinician trainees and expanding advanced practice clinicians' scope of practice to grow the abortion care workforce.[9]

Protecting the Abortion Workforce

Abortion care workers are frequently subjected to an onslaught of antiabortion harassment, intimidation, and violence.[2] The fatal shooting of Minnesota House Speaker Melissa Hortman and her husband Mark in June 2025 by an alleged antiabortion extremist with a suspected hitlist of 70 individuals including abortion providers, advocates, and prochoice politicians[10] is a tragic reminder of the pervasiveness of this violence.

Furthermore, ongoing attempts to repeal the federal Freedom of Access to Clinic Entrances Act[11] has heightened abortion providers' fears of increasingly dangerous threats to safety. Locally, city councilmembers in Carbondale, Illinois, enacted an ordinance establishing a 100-foot buffer zone around abortion clinics to limit exposure to protesters, which was later rescinded after a lawsuit by a local antiabortion group. In February 2025, the US Supreme Court declined to hear the antiabortion challenge to this policy,[12] suggesting that—for now—jurisdictions may successfully implement similar measures to protect abortion providers. Shield laws prohibiting out-of-state prosecution, professional discipline, and civil liability minimize legal risks to abortion providers caring for out-of-state patients; enacting shield laws and including telehealth abortion provision within their scope are additional measures to enhance the security of abortion providers.

CONCLUSION

In this post-*Dobbs* era, the role of abortion-protective states has become increasingly and critically important for abortion access nationwide. To that end, the analysis by Smith et al. contributes powerful evidence, demonstrating the increase in demand for care, particularly among out-of-state patients. We highlight important public health policy and practice implications spurred by their findings, including the opportunity for implementing policies at the state, community, and clinic levels to expand access to care and better meet the needs of abortion seekers nationally. Furthermore, we emphasize the urgent need to support clinics in abortion-protective settings, including prioritizing efforts to protect the health, well-being, and safety of the abortion workforce amid growing antiabortion violence. **AJPH**

CORRESPONDENCE

Correspondence should be sent to Sara K. Redd, 1518 Clifton Rd NE, Atlanta, GA 30322 (e-mail: skredd@emory.edu). Reprints can be ordered at https://www.ajph.org by clicking the "Reprints" link.

PUBLICATION INFORMATION

Full Citation: Redd SK, Filippa S, Luke AA, McMahon HV, Chew Murphy E. The opportunity of abortion-protective states in the post-*Dobbs* era: implications for public health policy and practice. *Am J Public Health.* 2026;116(3):326–328.

Acceptance Date: October 10, 2025.

DOI: https://doi.org/10.2105/AJPH.2025.308323

ORCID iDs:

Sara K. Redd https://orcid.org/0000-0002-2422-8937

Alina A. Luke https://orcid.org/0000-0002-6273-5219

Hayley V. McMahon https://orcid.org/0000-0003-4919-8612

CONTRIBUTORS

S. K. Redd conceptualized the editorial. S. K. Redd, S. Filippa, A. A. Luke, and H. V. McMahon drafted the editorial. E. Chew Murphy led the application of provider- and clinic-centered approaches. S. K. Redd and E. Chew Murphy revised the editorial. All authors reviewed and approved the final version.

ACKNOWLEDGMENTS

Work on this publication was funded in part by RISE through support from an anonymous foundation. S. K. Redd was supported in part by the Building Interdisciplinary Research Careers in Women's Health of the National Institutes of Health under award K12AR084234.

Note. The content is solely the responsibility of the authors and does not necessarily represent the official views of the National Institutes of Health.

CONFLICTS OF INTEREST

The authors have no conflicts of interest to disclose.

REFERENCES

1. Sabbath EL, McKetchnie SM, Arora KS, Buchbinder M. US obstetrician-gynecologists' perceived impacts of post-*Dobbs v Jackson* state abortion bans. *JAMA Netw Open.* 2024;7(1):e2352109. https://doi.org/10.1001/jamanetworkopen.2023.52109
2. National Abortion Federation. *NAF 2024 Violence & Disruption Report*. 2024. Available at: https://prochoice.org/our-work/provider-security/2024-naf-violence-disruption. Accessed September 8, 2025.
3. Berglas NF, Schroeder R, Kaller S, Stewart C, Upadhyay UD. Changes in availability of later abortion care before and after *Dobbs v Jackson Women's Health Organization*. *Obstet Gynecol.* 2025;145(1):e31–e36. https://doi.org/10.1097/AOG.0000000000005772
4. Dindinger E, Coleman-Minahan K, Sheeder J, Fang NZ. The impact of the SB 8 Texas abortion ban on pregnancy duration at time of abortion in a large volume Colorado clinic. *Contraception.* 2025;143:110731. https://doi.org/10.1016/j.contraception.2024.110731
5. Maddow-Zimet I, Philbin J, DoCampo I, Jones RK. Monthly Abortion Provision Study. August 21, 2025. Available at: https://osf.io/k4x7t. Accessed September 5, 2025.
6. Abortion Care Network. *Communities Need Clinics: 2024 Report*. 2024:35. Available at: https://abortioncarenetwork.org/wp-content/uploads/2024/12/CommunitiesNeedClinics2024_WEB-FINAL.pdf. Accessed September 8, 2025.
7. Weitz TA. Making sense of the economics of abortion in the United States. *Perspect Sex Reprod Health.* 2024;56(3):199–210. https://doi.org/10.1111/psrh.12288
8. Chowdhary P, Newton-Levinson A, Rochat R. "No one does this for the money or lifestyle": abortion providers' perspectives on factors affecting workforce recruitment and retention in the Southern United States. *Matern Child Health J.* 2022;26(6):1350–1357. https://doi.org/10.1007/s10995-021-03338-6
9. Illinois Department of Public Health. IDPH awards $2 million in training grants to 3 groups to improve reproductive health services. April 11, 2024. Available at: https://dph.illinois.gov/resource-center/news/2024/april/2024-04-11—idph-awards–2-million-in-training-grants-to-3-grou.html. Accessed September 8, 2025.
10. Karnowski S, Richer A, Seewer J. Minnesota shooting suspect had dozens of potential targets, prosecutors say. *Associated Press.* June 17, 2025. Available at: https://apnews.com/article/minnesota-lawmakers-shooting-dozens-targeted-d3d7866c09765fac088e6418e49ad811. Accessed October 2, 2025.
11. FACE Act Repeal Act of 2025. HR 589, 119th Cong, 2025–2026 sess (CR 2025).
12. *Coalition Life, Petitioner v City of Carbondale, Illinois.* US Supreme Court. Docket No. 24-57. 2024. Available at: https://www.supremecourt.gov/docket/docketfiles/html/public/24-57.html. Accessed September 8, 2025.

Reproductive Autonomy Restrictions as Collective Violence

N. Jeanie Santaularia Gomez, PhD, MPH, Krista Neumann, PhD, Maryam Tanveer, MPH, Kriszta Farkas, PhD, MPH, and Molly Altman, PhD, CNM, MPH

See also Abortion and Public Health Impact in Post-*Dobbs* Era, pp. 321–367.

In this essay, we argue that policies that intentionally or unintentionally restrict reproductive autonomy constitute an act of violence.

First, we discuss our guiding framework, highlighting the intersections between reproductive autonomy, reproductive justice, and violence. Second, we describe the importance of framing the restriction of reproductive autonomy as violence, emphasizing potential implications. Finally, we provide 3 illustrative examples of how governmental power—through the passage of laws—can both support and constrain reproductive autonomy across the life course: sex education, abortion restrictions, and parental leave policies. For each, we explain how the consequent harms overlap with those resulting from more traditional overt forms of violence.

By framing the loss of reproductive autonomy as a form of violence, we underscore its profound and far-reaching harms, demanding urgent recognition and response as a critical public health and human rights issue. (*Am J Public Health*. 2026;116(3):329–336. https://doi.org/10.2105/AJPH.2025.308276)

AJPH March 2026, Vol. 116, No. 3

Restrictions on reproductive autonomy—or the ability to make informed, independent decisions about one's reproductive health—are deeply embedded in US history and persist today, culminating most recently in renewed assaults on abortion rights. The 2022 *Dobbs v Jackson Women's Health Organization* US Supreme Court decision (*Dobbs*) overturned nearly 5 decades of federal protection for abortion access, effectively dismantling the legal precedent set by *Roe v Wade*. In the aftermath of *Dobbs*, 10 states passed constitutional amendments to protect abortion rights,[1] and 21 states have enacted a variety of protections for providers and patients.[2] However, numerous states have enacted bans or severe restrictions on abortion, thereby threatening reproductive rights across the nation. As of July 2025, 41 states had some type of abortion restriction in effect: 12 states have total or near-total abortion bans, 7 states permit abortion at varying gestational limits before 18 weeks of pregnancy, and 22 states permit abortion until viability or near viability as allowed pre-*Dobbs* (under *Roe v Wade*).[3]

In this essay, we argue that policies that intentionally or unintentionally restrict reproductive autonomy constitute an act of violence. First, we discuss our guiding framework; second, we describe the importance of framing the restriction of reproductive autonomy as violence; and, finally, we provide illustrative examples and explain how 3 specific policies restrict reproductive autonomy and result in physical or psychological harm. By framing the loss of reproductive autonomy as a form of violence, we underscore its profound and far-reaching harms, demanding urgent recognition and response as a critical public health and human rights issue.

GUIDING FRAMEWORK

This work is guided by the intersection of the defining elements of reproductive autonomy, reproductive justice, and violence. Reproductive autonomy is the entitlement of all people to shape their lives by making self-governing decisions regarding their reproductive health, regardless of their intersecting identities.[4] Reproductive health choices include but are not limited to whether to become pregnant (e.g., using contraception or birth control to prevent pregnancies) and the timing, number, context, and outcomes of pregnancies (e.g., deciding when to become pregnant, with whom to become pregnant, and whether to continue a pregnancy).

Reproductive justice[5] further broadens the scope of reproductive autonomy to encompass equitable access to reproductive health choices and quality of life when making these decisions and embeds it within a human rights framework.[5] Specifically, it is "the human right to maintain personal bodily autonomy, have children, not have children, and parent the children we have in safe and sustainable communities."[6] Structural factors such as education, racism, social class, environmental safety, social welfare, and immigration laws affect the ability of some individuals to make autonomous reproductive decisions. The harm that comes from the lack of power to determine one's own reproductive autonomy affects not only one's right to have or not to have children but also one's ability to support and parent children. In this essay, we use the lens of reproductive justice to help illustrate how loss of reproductive autonomy constitutes an act of violence.

Violence is defined by the World Health Organization (WHO) as,

> the intentional use of physical force or power, threatened or actual, against oneself, another person, or against a group or community, that either results in or has a high likelihood of resulting in injury, death, psychological harm, maldevelopment or deprivation.[7]

The WHO definition of violence has two key components. First, violence encompasses the "intentional use" of the act (physical force or power) itself, which is in contrast to unintentional acts such as accidental motor vehicle crashes. Importantly, the definition includes actions that are intentional, although the resulting harm may not be. This particular point was highlighted in the WHO world report on violence and health: "The presence of an intent to use force does not necessarily mean that there was an intent to cause harm."[7]

Second, the use of "power" in addition to "physical force" expands the definition to include the ability to influence or control the behavior of others to the extent that their well-being is harmed. Violence can be broken down into typologies categorized by the relationship between the perpetrator and victim (self-directed, interpersonal, collective violence) and further differentiated by the nature of the violent act (physical, sexual, psychological). Collective violence is typically committed by larger groups of individuals or states.

Guided by these 3 frameworks, we argue that restriction of reproductive autonomy through the intentional passing of federal, state, and local laws that prevent individuals from choosing how and when to have children results in profound harm to individuals and communities. These harms parallel those resulting from more traditional overt forms of violence; thus, by definition, the passage of these laws constitutes an act of collective violence.

FRAMING RESTRICTION OF REPRODUCTIVE AUTONOMY AS VIOLENCE

Simply, words matter. The framing of the structural restriction of reproductive rights as an act of violence underscores both the severity of its harms and the urgency for action. Naming an act as violent calls for a set of societal, legal, and ethical responses. The term "violence" serves as a powerful concept that influences our collective understanding of what is acceptable or unacceptable as a society. The defining of restriction of reproductive autonomy as violence also challenges the traditional and narrow view of violence as solely overt, brutal acts committed by individuals. It broadens the concept to include less visible—but equally harmful, if not more so, because of their widespread impact—uses of force and power by larger entities such as governments, institutions, and systems that shape the conditions under which individuals can make decisions about their reproductive lives.

Similar concepts of violence have been described in the literature at the interpersonal level, most notably obstetric violence.[8] Obstetric violence is typically defined as gender-based, individually mediated violence toward pregnant and birthing people, which can include mistreatment, disrespectful care, and abuse by health care providers and staff. Included as part of disrespectful care is loss of autonomy, which in this case is individuals not being provided the opportunity to make informed choices that best fit their needs.[9] Although often described as occurring at the interpersonal level, obstetric violence also encompasses systemic harms perpetrated by the health care system itself. For example, routine coercive interventions, withholding of clear information for informed decision-making, and the inability to act as a result of fear of legal repercussions represent a normalization of violence within medicalized maternity care.[10] In such cases, the institution's policies and culture—not just individual providers—are enacting the harm, which fits the definition of collective violence.[8]

Therefore, reframing legal restrictions of reproductive autonomy as violence is not only appropriate but warranted. It is important to frame restricting reproductive autonomy as collective or structural violence because, similar to obstetric violence, it is often normalized. Although it is intentional, it is often less overt, sometimes committed under the guise of religion or morality, and thus it may not be perceived as brutal and thereby violent.[11] Framing reproductive autonomy restriction as a form of violence highlights that it is a preventable act with important negative social[12] and health-related consequences[13] and thus necessitates a public health intervention.

ILLUSTRATIVE EXAMPLES

We examine 3 types of policies—sex education, abortion restrictions, and parental leave—that involve the use of multifaceted power to control reproductive autonomy across the life course. For each, we highlight how the resulting harms parallel those caused by more overt forms of violence. These illustrative examples demonstrate how policies can offer some degree of support for reproductive autonomy while simultaneously introducing barriers that prevent individuals from being able to make fully informed decisions about their bodies and futures, whether by design or as an unintended consequence. Each of these policies exists on a broad spectrum of influence, ranging from those that severely restrict autonomy (e.g., abstinence-only education, total abortion bans with limited exceptions, no parental leave) to those that actively support and expand individuals' ability to make informed, autonomous decisions about their reproductive lives. As with other definitions of violence, this wide spectrum of influence involves a similarly wide variation in impact.

In the sections to follow, we present arguments highlighting aspects of these 3 policies that meet the definition of violence, focusing on key exemplars within the policy spectrum. However, any violation of a human right, in this case reproductive policies that offer only piecemeal, time-limited, or conditional access to reproductive autonomy (whether through institutionalized withholding of information and medical procedures or confusing caveats and stipulations relating to access), is ultimately an act of violence.

Sex Education

Sex education in the United States has historically been shaped by political, religious, and cultural forces, resulting in wide variation across states and school districts. Today, sex education ranges from comprehensive, gender-inclusive evidence-based programs to abstinence-only curricula, also known as "sexual risk avoidance education."[14]

Comprehensive sex education, as implemented in some states, provides medically accurate, culturally competent, and gender-inclusive instruction that covers contraception, consent, and healthy relationships alongside information on abstinence.[15] Research consistently demonstrates that such programs lead to positive health outcomes, including reductions in intimate partner violence, healthy relationship development, prevention of child sexual abuse, improved social emotional learning, and reductions in sexual risk behaviors.[16]

By contrast, abstinence-only education remains the mandated approach in many states,[15] and an abstinence-only education or sexual risk avoidance education programs receive annual funding from the federal government ($8.8 million in fiscal year 2024).[17] These programs promote the idea that sex should occur only within marriage and discourage discussion of contraception and sexual health. Although sex education is essential for young people, abstinence-based education is a harmful approach that misconstrues and withholds key information. Research has shown that abstinence-only programs are ineffective in delaying sexual initiation, reducing risky sexual behaviors, and improving reproductive health outcomes.[18] Moreover, they are linked to misinformation, stigma, and increased vulnerability to sexual violence.[19] By denying youths access to medically accurate, comprehensive information about their own bodies and health, these programs systematically deprive them of the tools necessary to make informed decisions, thereby restricting their reproductive autonomy.

We posit that continued government funding of abstinence-only sex education—and indeed any program short of comprehensive, medically accurate, culturally competent, and gender-inclusive instruction—constitutes a form of collective violence because it is intentional use of power (through state policy and federally allocated dollars), threatened or actual (in this case actual), against a group or community (e.g., youths) that increases the likelihood of harmful outcomes including injury, death, psychological harm, maldevelopment, or deprivation. Historically, limited access to reproductive health education has contributed to cycles of unintended pregnancies, reproductive coercion, and constrained life opportunities, with disproportionate impacts for marginalized communities.[20] Furthermore, this is problematic because unintended pregnancy in adolescence is linked with poor maternal and infant physical and mental health outcomes as well as negative socioeconomic outcomes.[21]

In the digital age, misinformation about sex and reproductive health is widespread, making access to medically accurate sex education even more critical. From a reproductive justice perspective, withholding comprehensive information about one's sexual and reproductive health options is a violation of human rights—one that systematically undermines individuals' autonomy and well-being—thereby further supporting the notion that it is an act of collective violence.

Abortion Restrictions

Abortion restrictions in the United States have deep historical roots in systems of racial and gender-based oppression. Initially implemented to control the reproduction of enslaved Black people, suppress women's autonomy, and maintain White populations, these restrictions have long served as tools of reproductive control.[22] These efforts were further reinforced as mechanisms of coercion and subjugation by overt acts of violence such as rape and femicide.[22] Today, state-level restrictions on reproductive autonomy continue to be grounded in the exercise of power over marginalized populations, perpetuating dangerous gender norms and structural inequalities.

In the wake of the *Dobbs* decision, which removed constitutional protections for abortion, a surge in restrictive state-level antiabortion laws has created significant public health concerns.[23] This ruling has enabled states to completely ban and criminalize abortion, stripping pregnant-capable people of their bodily autonomy[23] and leading to widespread instances of forced pregnancies, that is, pregnancies that are unwanted or unintended yet carried to term because of legal, financial, or logistical barriers associated with abortion access.[24] The consequences of abortion restrictions extend beyond abortion itself to include constraining reproductive autonomy for those wishing to carry pregnancies to term, to access contraception, or to receive essential reproductive care.[25]

Pregnancy carries inherent risks.[26] Maternal mortality has been rising in recent years, with the US maternal mortality rate reaching 32.9 deaths per 100 000 live births in 2021, a stark increase from 20.1 in 2019.[27] These risks are disproportionately borne by Black birthing people, who in 2021 faced a maternal mortality rate of 69.9 deaths per 100 000 live births, 2.6 times the rate for White birthing people.[27] Beyond mortality, pregnancy increases the risk of hypertension, gestational diabetes, infections, and depression and anxiety.[26] Barriers to reproductive autonomy extend beyond pregnancy and childbirth; religiously affiliated hospitals frequently restrict access to reproductive autonomy by denying related procedures such as postdelivery tubal ligations,[28] thereby stripping pregnant-capable people of their autonomy to avoid risks associated with future pregnancy.

Abortion restrictions also exacerbate systemic health and socioeconomic disparities. Individuals denied an abortion are more likely to remain in relationships with abusive partners,[29] experience food insecurity,[12] and suffer long-term health problems.[30] Research shows that pregnant-capable people who were denied an abortion faced increased economic hardship, including lower credit scores, greater debt, and higher rates of bankruptcies and evictions.[31] Furthermore, restrictive state abortion laws are associated with increases in homicides related to intimate partner violence among women and girls of reproductive age.[32] Following *Dobbs*, an estimated 64 000 survivors of rape in abortion ban states faced rape-related pregnancies, with little or no access to legal abortion even in states with rape exceptions.[33] The burdens of forced pregnancy, childbirth, and child rearing all disproportionately affect pregnant-capable people of color, exacerbating existing racial and economic inequities.[34] All pregnant-capable individuals deserve the autonomy to choose whether to take on these burdens.

We posit that continued government support of the *Dobbs* decision constitutes a form of collective violence because it is the intentional use of state power through institutional mechanisms (e.g., state policies), threatened or actual (in this case actual), against a group or community (e.g., pregnant-capable people) that either results in or has a high likelihood of resulting in injury, death, psychological harm, maldevelopment, or deprivation. By restricting access to abortion and essential reproductive health care, these state-level laws systematically create conditions that increase the risk of injury, illness, and economic insecurity, thereby meeting the definition of violence and reinforcing a system of oppression. In line with reproductive justice, the right to have children, not have children, and parent those children in safe and sustainable environments is a fundamental human right.[5] Abortion restrictions violate this right, making them not just a public health crisis but an act of collective violence against pregnant-capable individuals.

Parental Leave Policies

The Family and Medical Leave Act (FMLA), signed into law in 1993, "is a federal law that guarantees job-protected, unpaid time off to eligible workers for qualifying reasons, such as bonding with a new child."[35] Although the FMLA is a critical step in recognizing the need for parental leave, it remains highly restrictive, insufficient, and unpaid, which exacerbates inequalities, particularly for marginalized populations.

First, the FMLA is highly restrictive, requiring that employees have worked for their employer for at least 1 year and completed 1250 hours of service during this time.[36] This contingency contributes to only 56% of US employees qualifying for the FMLA.[37]

Second, the FMLA is insufficient. Even for those who qualify, 12 weeks of unpaid leave often fall short of meeting the medical and developmental needs of both birthing parents and infants.[38] Typically, birthing parents' last visit to their medical provider is around 6 weeks postpartum. Often, however, self-reported recovery times from pregnancy, labor, and delivery are greater than that, with postpartum individuals reporting needing up to 1 year after delivery. Furthermore, parent–child bonding is imperative for healthy child development, with evidence supporting a minimum of 6 months—but ideally a full year—of dedicated time for caregiving.[39] Despite these needs, financial constraints force many parents to return to work far earlier than recommended: 1 in 4 employed birthing individuals return to work within 2 weeks of giving birth and nearly half by 6 weeks.[40]

Finally, and most notably, the FMLA is unpaid. A new child is incredibly expensive, costing upwards of $30 000 in the first year alone, excluding medical costs associated with the delivery itself.[41] For a household earning the US median income of approximately $80 000 in 2023,[41] taking 3 months of unpaid leave would reduce the annual income to approximately $50 000, leaving families with significantly less financial security to raise their new child and maintain household necessities. As a result, only families with sufficient savings or wealth can afford to take full advantage of the FMLA, reinforcing existing economic and racial inequities and contributing to a large share of parents returning to work earlier than recommended. Moreover, many jobs, particularly those held by women of color and individuals with lower educational attainment, do not qualify for FMLA protections at all, further marginalizing these workers.[42]

The existence of the FMLA—although a critical first step—has helped normalize the notion that limited, unpaid leave is an adequate societal response to caregiving needs. By establishing this as a baseline, it sets a low standard for how caregiving is valued in the United States, making it more difficult to advocate for more expansive, equitable leave policies.

Thirteen states and the District of Columbia have passed paid leave into law since 2004. Yet the United States remains the only high-income country without a federal paid parental leave policy, despite overwhelming evidence of its benefits.[43] By contrast, European countries mandate a minimum of 14 weeks of paid maternity leave, with many offering significantly more.[44] For example, Sweden provides 480 days of paid parental leave, and Germany offers up to 14 months of paid leave shared between parents.[44] These policies have been associated with better maternal and child health outcomes, stronger workforce retention, and reduced gender pay disparities.[44] In the United States, the lack of paid leave contributes to economic insecurity and adverse health outcomes, with one study showing 47% increased odds of infant rehospitalization and 51% increased odds of maternal rehospitalization by 21 months postpartum relative to women with paid leave.[43]

We posit that the FMLA, which normalizes insufficient, unpaid parental leave, constitutes a form of collective violence because it is the intentional use of power through institutional mechanisms (e.g., federal policy), threatened or actual (in this case actual), against a group or community (e.g., families) that is likely to result in harm, including injury, death, psychological harm, maldevelopment, or deprivation. From a reproductive justice perspective, the absence of a national paid parental leave policy is not simply an oversight; it is a structural failure that places economic and health burdens disproportionately on the most vulnerable parents and children, thereby meeting the definition of violence.

CONCLUSION

Violence extends beyond immediate physical harm; it encompasses the direct and downstream consequences that undermine an individual's psychological, social, political, and economic well-being. State and federal policies—whether enacted through local mandates, legislative statutes, or Supreme Court decisions—are violent when they systematically restrict civil liberties such as the right to privacy or when they limit individuals' economic, social, or political freedoms, resulting in wide-ranging negative consequences for entire communities. In this way, policies that restrict reproductive autonomy function as a form of collective violence, disproportionately harming those who are already most vulnerable and marginalized.

By reframing the implementation of policies that restrict reproductive autonomy as an act of collective violence, we can make more explicit their widespread and enduring harms. This shift in framing strengthens the case for policy change, expands access to information and services, and enriches public discourse by highlighting how state and federal regulations limiting reproductive rights have profound and far-reaching consequences: they not only have immediate health repercussions, but they also generate lasting intergenerational effects, entrench economic insecurity, exacerbate health disparities, and reinforce gender-based oppression. Within the specific context of restrictions on abortion rights, sexual education, and paid parental leave, the harm caused may be initially seen as finite (e.g., limited to reproductive health, only affecting individuals who have the capacity to reproduce) and perhaps even insignificant. On the contrary, such restrictions on reproductive autonomy have implications for everyone—all genders, all ages, all reproductive capacities—given how integral reproduction is to our society as a whole and its far-reaching impacts.

Our article centers how groups of individuals are violating a human right that is foundational for a thriving society, an act that by its very nature is violent and therefore necessitates a shift in how we frame public discourse and support affected communities. Thought leaders can draw from the wealth of knowledge that documents the harms of violence and how to support survivors to implement more expansive and innovative approaches to supporting bodily autonomy. For example, trauma-informed and survivor-centered interventions are well documented as a critical tool to prevent violence. By adopting this framework, society may be able to provide new and more effective forms of support in the current changing environment.

Importantly, from a public health perspective, this reframing serves as a necessary call to action, not only to mitigate harm but also to confront and dismantle the ideological foundations underpinning the control of women and pregnant-capable people within society. The violence and its downstream harms inflicted through the implementation of such policies are preventable and demand accountability from states and the federal government.

Just as we have mobilized public health responses to other forms of violence deemed public health crises, including gun violence, intimate partner violence, and child maltreatment,[45] recognizing restrictions on reproductive rights as collective violence demands a robust response. For example, the reframing of gun violence as a public health problem led to changes in funding priorities, resulting in increased investment in gun violence prevention research.[46] This, in turn, expanded knowledge about effective strategies to mitigate and prevent gun violence while raising public knowledge. This perspective shift challenges policymakers, health professionals, and advocates to actively counteract the harms inflicted by reproductive oppression (e.g., through policy changes) and affirm that reproductive autonomy is a fundamental component of health, equity, and human rights. AJPH

ABOUT THE AUTHORS

N. Jeanie Santaularia Gomez is with the Department of Epidemiology, School of Public Health, University of Washington, Seattle. Krista Neumann is with the Department of Pediatrics, School of Medicine, University of Washington. At the time of this writing, Maryam Tanveer was with the Department of Epidemiology, School of Public Health, University of Washington. Kriszta Farkas is with the Division of Epidemiology & Community Health, University of Minnesota, Minneapolis. Molly Altman is with the Department of Nursing, University of Hawaii at Manoa.

CORRESPONDENCE

Correspondence should be sent to N. Jeanie Santaularia Gomez, PhD, MPH, Hans Rosling Center for Population Health, 3980 15th Ave NE, Seattle, WA 98105 (e-mail: njsanta@uw.edu). Reprints can be ordered at http://www.ajph.org by clicking the "Reprints" link.

PUBLICATION INFORMATION

Full Citation: Santaularia Gomez NJ, Neumann K, Tanveer M, Farkas K, Altman M. Reproductive autonomy restrictions as collective violence. *Am J Public Health*. 2026;116(3):329–336.

Acceptance Date: August 16, 2025.

DOI: https://doi.org/10.2105/AJPH.2025.308276

ORCID iDs:

N. Jeanie Santaularia Gomez https://orcid.org/0000-0002-2861-7606

Krista Neumann https://orcid.org/0000-0002-7527-4482

Maryam Tanveer https://orcid.org/0009-0001-8559-0702

Kriszta Farkas https://orcid.org/0000-0003-1605-580X

Molly Altman https://orcid.org/0000-0002-0453-0469

CONTRIBUTORS

All of the authors made substantial contributions to drafting the work or revising it critically for important intellectual content.

ACKNOWLEDGMENTS

Partial support for this research came from the University of Washington Center for Studies in Demography & Ecology, whose funders include the Eunice Kennedy Shriver National Institute of Child Health and Human Development (NICHD; research infrastructure grant P2C HD042828) and multiple units at the university: the College of Arts

& Sciences, Office of Research, eSciences Institute, Evans School of Public Policy, College of Built Environments, School of Public Health, Foster School of Business, and School of Social Work. Additional partial support was provided through NICHD grant T32HD057822.

Note. The content is solely the responsibility of the authors and does not necessarily represent the official views of the National Institutes of Health.

CONFLICTS OF INTEREST

There are no conflicts of interest.

HUMAN PARTICIPANT PROTECTION

This study did not involve human participants.

REFERENCES

1. Felix M, Sobel L. A continuing saga: ending abortion restrictions in states with constitutional protections. Available at: https://www.kff.org/policy-watch/a-continuing-saga-ending-abortion-restrictions-in-states-with-constitutional-protections. Accessed August 15, 2025.
2. McCann A, Walker AS. Tracking abortion laws across the country. Available at: https://www.nytimes.com/interactive/2024/us/abortion-laws-roe-v-wade.html. Accessed August 15, 2025.
3. Guttmacher Institute. State bans on abortion throughout pregnancy. Available at: https://www.guttmacher.org/state-policy/explore/state-policies-abortion-bans. Accessed June 22, 2025.
4. Chalasani S, Diop N, Filmer-Wilson E, Liang M, Sharafi L. My body is my own: claiming the right to autonomy and self-determination. Available at: https://www.unfpa.org/sowp-2021. Accessed September 24, 2024.
5. Davis DA. *Reproductive Injustice: Racism, Pregnancy, and Premature Birth.* New York University Press; 2019.
6. Sister Song. Reproductive justice. Available at: https://www.sistersong.net/reproductive-justice. Accessed June 22, 2025.
7. Krug EG, Mercy JA, Dahlberg LL, Zwi AB. The world report on violence and health. Available at: https://iris.who.int/server/api/core/bitstreams/a25476ed-8585-47f3-986e-9d0e7f5e9f1b/content. Accessed June 22, 2025.
8. Pickles C. 'Everything is obstetric violence now': identifying the violence in 'obstetric violence' to strengthen socio-legal reform efforts. *Oxf J Leg Stud.* 2024;44(3):616–644. https://doi.org/10.1093/ojls/gqae016
9. Vedam S, Stoll K, McRae DN, et al. Patient-led decision making: measuring autonomy and respect in Canadian maternity care. *Patient Educ Couns.* 2019;102(3):586–594. https://doi.org/10.1016/j.pec.2018.10.023
10. Buchbinder M, Sabbath EL. Reproductive healthcare after *Dobbs*: rethinking obstetric harm in the United States. Available at: https://www.tandfonline.com/doi/full/10.1080/01459740.2024.2438034. Accessed June 22, 2025.
11. Law, Rights, and Religion Project. A religious right to abortion: legal history and analysis. Available at: https://scholarship.law.columbia.edu/gender_sexuality_law/18. Accessed June 22, 2025.
12. Foster DG, Biggs MA, Ralph L, Gerdts C, Roberts S, Glymour MM. Socioeconomic outcomes of women who receive and women who are denied wanted abortions in the United States. *Am J Public Health.* 2022;112(9):1290–1296. https://doi.org/10.2105/AJPH.2017.304247
13. Bossick AS, Williams EC, Painter I, Katon JG. Association of reproductive autonomy and rates of state-level racialized disparities in preterm birth and low birthweight. *Health Equity.* 2023;7(1):497–505. https://doi.org/10.1089/heq.2023.0060
14. Eisenstein Z. Why we need to avoid sexual risk avoidance. Available at: https://siecus.org/why-we-need-to-avoid-sexual-risk-avoidance/, https://news.siecus.org/why-we-need-to-avoid-sexual-risk-avoidance. Accessed March 28, 2025.
15. SIECUS. State profiles. Available at: https://siecus.org/stateprofiles. Accessed April 4, 2025.
16. Goldfarb ES, Lieberman LD. Three decades of research: the case for comprehensive sex education. *J Adolesc Health.* 2021;68(1):13–27. https://doi.org/10.1016/j.jadohealth.2020.07.036
17. Grants.gov. Title V competitive sexual risk avoidance education. Available at: https://grants.gov/search-results-detail/354008. Accessed March 28, 2025.
18. Heels S. The impact of abstinence-only sex education programs in the United States on adolescent sexual outcomes. Available at: https://scholars.unh.edu/cgi/viewcontent.cgi?article=1114&context=perspectives. Accessed March 28, 2025.
19. Santelli JS, Kantor LM, Grilo SA, et al. Abstinence-only-until-marriage: an updated review of US policies and programs and their impact. *J Adolesc Health.* 2017;61(3):273–280. https://doi.org/10.1016/j.jadohealth.2017.05.031
20. Sutton MY, Anachebe NF, Lee R, Skanes H. Racial and ethnic disparities in reproductive health services and outcomes, 2020. *Obstet Gynecol.* 2021;137(2):225–233. https://doi.org/10.1097/AOG.0000000000004224
21. Leftwich HK, Alves MVO. Adolescent pregnancy. *Pediatr Clin North Am.* 2017;64(2):381–388. https://doi.org/10.1016/j.pcl.2016.11.007
22. Goodwin M. The racist history of abortion and midwifery bans. Available at: https://www.aclu.org/news/racial-justice/the-racist-history-of-abortion-and-midwifery-bans. Accessed July 15, 2023.
23. Schreiber CA, Khabele D, Gehrig PA. The Dobbs v Jackson Women's Health Organization Supreme Court decision—concerns, challenges, and consequences for health care. *JAMA Surg.* 2023;158(3):229–230. https://doi.org/10.1001/jamasurg.2022.5714
24. Ananat EO, Gruber J, Levine P, Staiger D. Abortion and selection. Available at: https://repository.wellesley.edu/object/ir94. Accessed July 15, 2023.
25. Paltrow LM, Harris LH, Marshall MF. Beyond abortion: the consequences of overturning Roe. *Am J Bioeth.* 2022;22(8):3–15. https://doi.org/10.1080/15265161.2022.2075965
26. Centers for Disease Control and Prevention. Pregnancy complications. Available at: https://www.cdc.gov/maternal-infant-health/pregnancy-complications/index.html. Accessed March 28, 2025.
27. National Center for Health Statistics. Maternal mortality rates in the United States, 2022. Available at: https://www.cdc.gov/nchs/data/hestat/maternal-mortality/2022/maternal-mortality-rates-2022.htm. Accessed March 28, 2025.
28. Stulberg DB, Hoffman Y, Dahlquist IH, Freedman LR. Tubal ligation in Catholic hospitals: a qualitative study of ob-gyns' experiences. *Contraception.* 2014;90(4):422–428. https://doi.org/10.1016/j.contraception.2014.04.015
29. Roberts SC, Biggs MA, Chibber KS, Gould H, Rocca CH, Foster DG. Risk of violence from the man involved in the pregnancy after receiving or being denied an abortion. *BMC Med.* 2014;12(1):144. https://doi.org/10.1186/s12916-014-0144-z
30. Gerdts C, Dobkin L, Foster DG, Schwarz EB. Side effects, physical health consequences, and mortality associated with abortion and birth after an unwanted pregnancy. *Womens Health Issues.* 2016;26(1):55–59. https://doi.org/10.1016/j.whi.2015.10.001
31. Miller S, Wherry L, Foster D. The economic consequences of being denied an abortion. Available at: https://papers.ssrn.com/abstract=3611484. Accessed January 8, 2025.
32. Wallace ME, Stoecker C, Sauter S, Vilda D. States' abortion laws associated with intimate partner violence–related homicide of women and girls in the US, 2014–20. *Health Aff (Millwood).* 2024;43(5):682–690. https://doi.org/10.1377/hlthaff.2023.01098
33. Dickman SL, White K, Himmelstein DU, Lupez E, Schrier E, Woolhandler S. Rape-related pregnancies in the 14 US states with total abortion bans. *JAMA Intern Med.* 2024;184(3):330–332. https://doi.org/10.1001/jamainternmed.2024.0014
34. Girardi G, Longo M, Bremer AA. Social determinants of health in pregnant individuals from underrepresented, understudied, and underreported populations in the United States. *Int J Equity Health.* 2023;22(1):186. https://doi.org/10.1186/s12939-023-01963-x
35. US Department of Labor. Family and Medical Leave Act. Available at: https://www.dol.gov/general/topic/benefits-leave/fmla. Accessed March 28, 2025.
36. US Department of Labor. FMLA leave for birth, placement, bonding, or to care for a child with a serious health condition on the basis of an "in loco parentis" relationship. Available at: https://www.dol.gov/agencies/whd/fact-sheets/28B-fmla-in-loco-parentis. Accessed March 28, 2025.
37. US Department of Labor. Employee and worksite perspectives of the Family and Medical Leave Act: results from the 2018 surveys. Available at: https://www.dol.gov/sites/dolgov/files/OASP/evaluation/pdf/WHD_FMLA2018SurveyResults_FinalReport_Aug2020.pdf. Accessed March 28, 2025.
38. Rossin M. The effects of maternity leave on children's birth and infant health outcomes in the United States. *J Health Econ.* 2011;30(2):221–239. https://doi.org/10.1016/j.jhealeco.2011.01.005
39. US Department of Labor. Taking leave from work for birth, placement, and bonding with a child under the FMLA. Available at: https://www.dol.gov/agencies/whd/fact-sheets/28q-taking-leave-for-birth-placement-child. Accessed March 28, 2025.
40. Lerner S. The real war on families: why the US needs paid leave now. Available at: https://inthesetimes.com/article/the-real-war-on-families. Accessed March 28, 2025.

41. Davis M, Shepard D. It costs $297,674 to raise a child over 18 years. Available at: https://www.lendingtree.com/debt-consolidation/raising-a-child-study. Accessed April 4, 2025.
42. Vohra-Gupta S, Kim Y, Cubbin C. Systemic Racism and the Family Medical Leave Act (FMLA): using critical race theory to build equitable family leave policies. *J Racial Ethn Health Disparities*. 2021; 8(6):1482–1491. https://doi.org/10.1007/s40615-020-00911-7
43. Jou J, Kozhimannil KB, Abraham JM, Blewett LA, McGovern PM. Paid maternity leave in the United States: associations with maternal and infant health. *Matern Child Health J*. 2018;22(2):216–225. https://doi.org/10.1007/s10995-017-2393-x
44. Strang L, Broeks M. Maternity leave policies. *Rand Health Q*. 2017;6(4):9.
45. American Public Health Association. Violence is a public health issue: public health is essential to understanding and treating violence in the US. Available at: https://www.apha.org/policies-and-advocacy/public-health-policy-statements/policy-database/2019/01/28/violence-is-a-public-health-issue. Accessed April 4, 2025.
46. American Public Health Association. APHA advocacy fact sheet for gun violence prevention. Available at: https://www.apha.org/getcontentasset/962debd2-5945-40fb-ab71-4239076c5e30/7ca0dc9d-611d-46e2-9fd3-26a4c03ddcbb/200221_gun_violence_fact_sheet.pdf?language=en. Accessed June 22, 2025.

Changes in Facility-Based Abortion Care Among Texas Resident Minors and Young Adults After a 2021 Abortion Ban: September 2020–May 2022

Kari White, PhD, MPH, Gracia Sierra, PhD, MA, Brooke Whitfield, PhD, Kristina Tocce, MD, MPH, Samuel L. Dickman, MD, and Vinita Goyal, MD, MPH

See also Abortion and Public Health Impact in Post-*Dobbs* Era, pp. 321–367.

Objectives. To compare changes in the number of facility-based abortions among Texas residents in different age groups following the state's 2021 law prohibiting abortion after detection of embryonic cardiac activity.

Methods. We obtained data from Texas and 6 surrounding states on Texas residents' age at abortion from state vital statistics and data provided directly by out-of-state abortion facilities. Using negative binomial regression, we estimated the percentage change in abortions before (September 2020–May 2021) and after (September 2021–May 2022) the law went into effect.

Results. After the law's implementation, total (in-state and out-of-state) facility-based abortions decreased by 26.1% (95% confidence interval [CI] = −32.7%, −18.8%) among Texans younger than 18 years, by 19.6% (95% CI = −21.4%, −17.7%) among young adult Texans aged 18 to 24 years, and by 17.0% (95% CI = −19.1%, −14.8%) among Texans aged 25 to 29 years.

Conclusions. Texas's law disproportionately affected access to facility-based abortion care among Texans aged 24 years and younger.

Public Health Implications. State laws prohibiting abortions in early pregnancy disproportionately affect young people's reproductive autonomy, likely by compounding long-standing financial and logistical barriers to facility-based care. (*Am J Public Health*. 2026;116(3):337–340. https://doi.org/10.2105/AJPH.2025.308289)

AJPH March 2026, Vol. 116, No. 3

On September 1, 2021, Texas implemented Senate Bill 8 (SB8), which prohibited abortion upon detection of embryonic cardiac activity—which occurs approximately 5 to 6 weeks after a pregnant person's last menstrual period. Following SB8's implementation, the total number of facility-based abortions that Texas residents obtained in Texas and surrounding states decreased significantly.[1] Compared with pregnant Texans aged 25 years and older, those younger than 18 years (i.e., minors) and those aged 18 to 24 years (i.e., young adults) may have been less likely to obtain facility-based care following bans on abortion in early pregnancy because of social, financial, and logistical barriers that disproportionately affect young people.[2–5] However, few studies have reported on age group–specific changes in total abortions after recent bans have gone into effect.[6]

In this analysis, we assessed changes in the number of abortions among Texas residents younger than 25 years compared with residents aged 25 years and older following implementation of SB8. We also examined out-of-state travel patterns according to state parental involvement requirements for minors (e.g., parental consent), which create additional barriers to care.[7]

METHODS

For the period September 2020 through May 2021 (before SB8's implementation), we obtained data on Texas residents' age at abortion from publicly available state vital statistics data and age group–specific totals provided by state health departments in Texas and 6 surrounding states (Appendix, available as a supplement to the online version of this article at http://www.ajph.org). Age group–specific information on Texans who obtained abortions in Arkansas and Kansas before SB8 was not available; we estimated this using information from each state's 2020 vital statistics report on the age distribution of all abortions and applied that distribution to the reported Texas resident total. For September 2021 through May 2022 (after the law's implementation), we used state health department data for Texas, Colorado, and Louisiana. Additionally, all abortion facilities in Arkansas and Oklahoma provided individual-level data on Texas residents; in Kansas and New Mexico, high-volume providers in each area of the state with abortion facilities (8 of 11 total facilities) provided individual-level data, thereby including the majority of Texas resident abortions.[1] Focusing on the 9-month periods between September and May enabled us to minimize the suppression of small values from any 1 state, account for abortion seasonality, and isolate changes associated with SB8 before Oklahoma abortion facilities suspended services in May 2022.

We calculated the number of Texas resident in-state, out-of-state, and total abortions by age group before and after SB8. We used negative binomial regression and Stata version 18 (StataCorp LP, College Station, TX) to estimate age group–specific percentage change for in-state, out-of-state, and total abortions after SB8 compared with before. In models including data from all age groups, we used age group × period interactions to assess whether changes among minors and young adults were significantly different from changes among those aged 25 to 29 years. Given the short time period for the study, we assumed a stable population and did not include a population offset. We considered 2-sided *P* less than .05 significant.

We used the χ^2 test to compare the percentage of minors who traveled to states with and without parental involvement requirements (consent or notification) before and after SB8, when minors' chances were low of obtaining in-state care without parental involvement (i.e., via judicial bypass) before detectable embryonic cardiac activity. Of the 6 surrounding states, only New Mexico did not require parental involvement, but facilities in other states were closer for residents in most Texas cities.[8]

RESULTS

Comparing the periods before and after SB8, the number of in-state facility-based abortions decreased among Texas minors (from 954 to 385), young adult Texans (from 15 422 to 8306), and Texans aged 25 to 29 years (from 12 149 to 7077; Table 1). The percentage decrease among minors (−59.6%; 95% confidence interval [CI] = −64.1%, −54.6%) and young adults (−46.1%; 95% CI = −47.6%, −44.7%) was significantly greater than the decrease among those aged 25 to 29 years (−41.7%; 95% CI = −43.4%, −40.0%; for age × period interactions: $P < .001$). The number of Texas minors who obtained out-of-state abortions increased from 62 before SB8 to 366 after SB8, from 834 to 4762 among young adult Texans, and from 577 to 3489 among Texans aged 25 to 29 years; the percentage change among minors and young adults was not significantly different from the percentage change among Texans aged 25 to 29 years ($P > .05$).

Total (combined in-state and out-of-state) facility-based abortions decreased 26.1% (95% CI = −32.7%, −18.8%) after SB8 among Texas resident minors, compared with a 17.0% (95% CI = −19.1%, −14.8%) decrease among Texans aged 25 to 29 years (age × period interaction: $P = .02$). Among young adult Texans, total facility-based abortions declined by 19.6% (95% CI = −21.4%, −17.7%) after SB8 ($P = .07$).

After SB8, 64% (234/366) of Texas minors obtained out-of-state abortion care in states with parental involvement requirements, compared with 53% (33/62) before SB8 ($P = .11$).

DISCUSSION

SB8 was associated with larger decreases in in-state facility-based abortions among Texas minors and young adult Texans compared with Texans aged 25 to 29 years. Before widespread implementation of abortion bans, young people faced unique barriers to abortion care.[4] That Texans younger than 25 years were less likely to obtain in-state care may be related to the challenges of overcoming multiple barriers before embryonic cardiac activity could be detected, for example, not recognizing pregnancy early, not knowing where to obtain an abortion,

TABLE 1— Number and Percentage Change in Facility-Based Abortions Obtained by Texas Residents in Texas and Out of State After Implementation of SB8, by Age Group: September 2020–May 2022

Age, y	Before SB8 (September 2020–May 2021), No. Abortions	After SB8 (September 2021–May 2022), No. Abortions	% Change (95% CI)[a]
Texas facilities			
< 18	954	385	−59.6 (−64.1, −54.6)
18–24	15 422	8 306	−46.1 (−47.6, −44.7)
25–29	12 149	7 077	−41.7 (−43.4, −40.0)
30–34	8 284	4 776	−42.3 (−44.4, −40.3)
≥ 35	5 912	3 459	−41.5 (−43.9, −39.0)
Out-of-state facilities[b]			
< 18	62	366	590.3 (451.0, 772.7)
18–24	834	4 762	571.0 (530.5, 614.6)
25–29	577	3 489	604.7 (553.7, 660.4)
30–34	334	2 273	680.5 (606.7, 763.4)
≥ 35	222	1 585	714.0 (620.4, 821.6)
Total			
< 18	1 016	751	−26.1 (−32.7, −18.8)
18–24	16 256	13 068	−19.6 (−21.4, −17.7)
25–29	12 726	10 566	−17.0 (−19.1, −14.8)
30–34	8 618	7 049	−18.2 (−20.7, −15.6)
≥ 35	6 134	5 044	−17.8 (−20.8, −14.6)

Note. CI = confidence interval; SB8 = Texas Senate Bill 8. We obtained data on Texas residents' age at abortion from publicly available state vital statistics data and age group–specific totals provided by state health departments in Texas and 6 surrounding states.
[a]We estimated % changes and 95% CIs from negative binomial regression models, including all age groups and age group × period interactions.
[b]Out-of-state facilities were located in Arkansas, Colorado, Kansas, Louisiana, New Mexico, and Oklahoma.

having to disclose their pregnancy to family members to travel and pay for care, and experiencing difficulties independently making these arrangements.[2,4,5,9]

Our findings further suggest that restrictive abortion laws disproportionately affect minors, who had the largest decrease in total facility-based abortions as well as greater increases in births after SB8's implementation.[10] These outcomes could be related, in part, to parental involvement laws that were in place in Texas and most surrounding states when SB8 was in effect. Minors who did not have parental consent were unlikely to obtain a judicial bypass and secure in-state care before detectable embryonic cardiac activity. Although most minors obtained care in states with parental involvement requirements after SB8, they may have done so because these facilities were closer to Texas's major metropolitan areas.[8] Parental involvement requirements also create financial and logistical obstacles for families and may delay care.[7,11]

A limitation of this study is that we did not obtain data from all out-of-state facilities, and some abortions may not be reported to state health departments; however, our data included the majority of abortions.[1] We also lacked information on gestational duration that could have provided insights into SB8's impact on care delays and people's need to travel to states that provide abortion later in pregnancy.

PUBLIC HEALTH IMPLICATIONS

Since the June 2022 Supreme Court decision in *Dobbs v Jackson Women's Health Org.* (597 US 215), 18 states have implemented laws that either prohibit abortion entirely or prohibit abortion after approximately 6 weeks' gestation; laws are currently in effect in 16 states. These restrictions may make it especially difficult for young people facing long travel distances to obtain abortion care—difficulties that could be greater for those younger than 18 years because some states have proposed or implemented laws restricting minors' out-of-state travel for abortion.[12] To support young people's reproductive autonomy, additional research is needed on their sources of abortion information to tailor efforts that ensure that they have accurate knowledge about how and where to obtain abortion care and how to access the financial, logistical, and legal support that they need.[5] States where abortion remains legal could remove parental involvement laws so minors can obtain confidential care, as professional medical associations recommend.[11] AJPH

ABOUT THE AUTHORS

Kari White and Gracia Sierra are with Resound Research for Reproductive Health, Austin, TX. Brooke Whitfield was with the Department of Sociology, University of Texas at Austin at the time of the study. Kristina Tocce is with Planned Parenthood of the Rocky Mountains, Denver, CO. Samuel L. Dickman is with Planned Parenthood of Montana, Billings, MT. Vinita Goyal is with Alamo Women's Clinic of Albuquerque, Albuquerque, NM.

CORRESPONDENCE

Correspondence should be sent to Kari White, 3908 Ave B, Austin, TX 78751 (e-mail: kariwhite@resoundrh.org). Reprints can be ordered at https://www.ajph.org by clicking the "Reprints" link.

PUBLICATION INFORMATION

Full Citation: White K, Sierra G, Whitfield B, Tocce K, Dickman SL, Goyal V. Changes in facility-based abortion care among Texas resident minors and young adults after a 2021 abortion ban: September 2020–May 2022. *Am J Public Health*. 2026;116(3): 337–340.

Acceptance Date: September 7, 2025.

DOI: https://doi.org/10.2105/AJPH.2025.308289

ORCID iD:
Samuel L. Dickman https://orcid.org/0000-0003-3126-786X

CONTRIBUTORS

K. White wrote the initial draft of the article. K. White and G. Sierra analyzed the data. K. White, K. Tocce, and V. Goyal acquired the data. K. White and S. L. Dickman conceptualized and designed the study. G. Sierra and B. Whitfield contributed to data management. All authors interpreted the data, critically reviewed the article, and approved the final version.

ACKNOWLEDGMENTS

This research was supported by grants from the Collaborative for Gender + Reproductive Equity (grant G-21-2122854), Jacob & Terese Hershey Foundation, and an anonymous private foundation.

Note. The funders had no role in the design and conduct of the study; collection, management, analysis, and interpretation of the data; preparation, review, or approval of the article; or decision to submit for publication. The findings and conclusions in this article are those of the authors and do not necessarily reflect the views of the funders or Planned Parenthood Federation of America, Inc.

CONFLICTS OF INTEREST

S. L. Dickman was a named plaintiff in the case *Planned Parenthood of Montana v State of Montana*, a lawsuit challenging abortion restrictions in Montana. The other authors have no conflicts of interest relevant to this article to disclose.

HUMAN PARTICIPANT PROTECTION

The University of Texas at Austin institutional review board approved study procedures.

REFERENCES

1. White K, Sierra G, Lerma K, et al. Association of Texas' 2021 ban on abortion in early pregnancy with the number of facility-based abortions in Texas and surrounding states. *JAMA*. 2022; 328(20):2048–2055. https://doi.org/10.1001/jama.2022.20423
2. Osborne C, Ankrum N. "Mom, I'm pregnant": The adolescent pregnancy reveal. *Soc Serv Rev*. 2020; 94(2):339–372. https://doi.org/10.1086/708749
3. Guttmacher Institute. Minors' access to abortion care. August 28, 2025. Available at: https://www.guttmacher.org/state-policy/explore/parental-involvement-minors-abortions. Accessed October 15, 2025.
4. Chiu DW, Braccia A, Jones RK. Characteristics and circumstances of adolescents obtaining abortions in the United States. *Int J Environ Res Public Health*. 2024;21(4):477. https://doi.org/10.3390/ijerph21040477
5. Vear K, Esbrook E, Padley E, Maslowsky J, Allison B, Hoopes A. "Time, money and support": adolescents and young adults' perceived social and logistical support needs for safe abortion care. *Contraception*. 2023;126:110128. https://doi.org/10.1016/j.contraception.2023.110128
6. Stevenson A. Decline in abortions by age group in the first six months of Texas Senate Bill 8 enforcement. *SocArXiv Papers*. 2022. Available at: https://doi.org/10.31235/osf.io/c5sdw. Accessed June 21, 2025.
7. White K, Narasimhan S, Hartwig SA, et al. Parental involvement policies for minors seeking abortion in the Southeast and quality of care. *Sex Res Soc Policy*. 2022;19(1):264–272. https://doi.org/10.1007/s13178-021-00539-0
8. White K, Vizcarra E, Palomares L, Dane'el A, Beasley A, Ogburn T. Initial impacts of Texas' Senate Bill 8 on abortions in Texas and at out-of-state facilities. October 2021. Available at: https://sites.utexas.edu/txpep/files/2021/10/initial-impacts-SB8-TxPEP-brief.pdf. Accessed March 7, 2024.
9. Ralph LJ, Foster DG, Barar RE, Rocca CH. Home pregnancy test use and timing of pregnancy confirmation among people seeking health care. *Contraception*. 2022;107(3):10–16. https://doi.org/10.1016/j.contraception.2021.10.006
10. University of Houston, Institute for Research on Women, Gender and Sexuality. Texas & Harris County reproductive health update: 2022 fertility rates, post 2021 six-week abortion ban. January 2024. Available at: https://www.uh.edu/class/ws/irwgs/_docs/2024/56999-ws-abortion-ban-report-v5.pdf. Accessed October 15, 2025.
11. American Academy of Pediatrics, Committee on Adolescence. The adolescent's right to confidential care when considering abortion. *Pediatrics*. 2022;150(3):e2022058780. https://doi.org/10.1542/peds.2022-058780
12. Rogers S. A patchwork nation: abortion laws and access challenges. October 31, 2024. Available at: https://www.billtrack50.com/info/blog/a-patchwork-nation-abortion-laws-and-access-challenges. Accessed June 1, 2025.

The Association Between State Gestational Age Limit Abortion Laws and Severe Maternal Morbidity: United States, 2010–2022

Nicole Siegal, PhD, and Aparna Soni, PhD

See also Abortion and Public Health Impact in Post-*Dobbs* Era, pp. 321–367.

Objectives. To investigate the association between state gestational age limit abortion laws, which restrict abortions after a specific point in pregnancy, and severe maternal morbidity (SMM) hospitalization rates in the United States.

Methods. We used a difference-in-differences approach and hospitalizations data measured annually at the state level from 2010 to 2022 for 47 states. All models included state covariates and state and year fixed effects, which provided plausibly causal estimates of the effect of gestational age limits on SMM rates.

Results. Any law that prohibited abortion on the basis of gestational age increased SMM rates by 7.67 (95% confidence interval [CI] = 1.55, 13.80) per 10 000 patients. This was equal to a 10.5% increase in SMM rates compared with baseline levels. The effects were driven by older patients, hospitalizations paid for by public payers, safety net hospitals, and patients living in low-income communities. Conversely, increasing the gestational age limit by 1 week (expanding abortion access) reduced the SMM rate by 0.28 (95% CI = −0.568, 0.002) per 10 000 patients.

Conclusions. Restricting access to abortion care increases the risk of SMM, particularly among older women and those of lower socioeconomic status. (*Am J Public Health*. 2026;116(3):341–344. https://doi.org/10.2105/AJPH.2025.308291)

AJPH March 2026, Vol. 116, No. 3

Severe maternal morbidity (SMM), which includes unexpected outcomes of labor and delivery that can result in substantial short-term and long-term health consequences, is rising in the United States and affects more than 35 000 women each year (Figure A, available as a supplement to the online version of this article at http://www.ajph.org). Meanwhile, women's access to abortion is decreasing because of numerous changes to the laws, including state-level gestational age limits, which restrict abortions after a specific point in pregnancy.[1] Between 2010 and 2022, 27 states decreased their gestational age limit (thereby reducing abortion access) by an average of 8 weeks, with 19 states prohibiting abortion after 20 weeks.[2] After the 2022 Supreme Court decision in *Dobbs v Jackson Women's Health Organization* (*Dobbs*; 597 US 215) eliminated federal protection of abortion rights, several states implemented even stricter gestational limits, banning abortion as early as 6 weeks (Appendix A, available as a supplement to the online version of this article at http://www.ajph.org).

A substantial body of research shows that gestational age limits can increase birth complications,[3] increase maternal and infant deaths,[4,5] and affect women's fertility decisions, health, and economic outcomes.[6–10] It is also plausible that gestational age limits on abortion may increase SMM by forcing women to carry risky pregnancies to term and increasing complications from unsafe abortions, but there is little empirical research on this topic.

This study fills that gap by estimating the association between gestational age limits and SMM from 2010 to 2022, which primarily covers the pre-*Dobbs* era. We used a difference-in-differences approach using variation in the presence and severity of gestational age limits across states and over time. Our findings contribute to the growing literature highlighting the adverse effects of abortion restrictions on maternal health.

METHODS

We obtained data on SMM from Healthcare Cost and Utilization Project (HCUP) Fast Stats, which provides state-level summary statistics on the number of in-hospital deliveries involving SMM each year between 2010 and 2022. We defined our main outcome variable as the rate of SMM per 10 000 in-hospital deliveries. HCUP provides this rate for the overall population as well as by select patient and hospital characteristics, including age group, income quartile, and expected payer. (See Appendix B [available as a supplement to the online version of this article at http://www.ajph.org] for additional details on the HCUP Fast Stats data.) We obtained data on state-level abortion laws from the Guttmacher Institute's "Overview of Abortion Laws" (Table A, available as a supplement to the online version of this article at http://www.ajph.org). We collected additional data on state covariates from the US Census Bureau and the Bureau of Labor Statistics.

We estimated difference-in-differences regression models for our main specification to capture the association between state gestational age limit laws and SMM rates. We conducted the statistical analyses using Stata version 19 (StataCorp LP, College Station, TX). Our models controlled for state-level economic and demographic characteristics, state fixed effects, and year fixed effects. We clustered SEs at the state level. Our first specification defined gestational age limit as a binary variable equal to 1 for any state-year observation in which a gestational age limit was present, and zero if not. Our second specification defined the law by using a continuous variable that was equal to the specific gestational week at which abortion is prohibited.

RESULTS

Figure A shows that SMM rates increased by nearly 45%: from 69.8 hospitalizations per 10 000 in-hospital deliveries in 2010 to 101.1 by 2021. Much of this increase happened during the COVID-19 pandemic.

Table 1 presents our difference-in-differences regression results. The table shows that the presence of any gestational age limit restriction increased the rate of SMM by 7.67 (95% confidence interval [CI] = 1.55, 13.80) per 10 000 deliveries. Relative to the baseline rate of 73.4, this represents a 10.5% increase. Our event study model shows that prelaw trends were not statistically significantly different between states with and those without restrictions, which supports the parallel trends assumption, a key assumption of the difference-in-differences model (Figure B, available as a supplement to the online version of this article at http://www.ajph.org).

Table 1, which presents results for the specific gestational week at which abortion became prohibited, shows that a 1-week increase in the age limit (i.e., more lenient law) was associated with a decrease in the SMM rate of 0.282 per 10 000 deliveries (95% CI = −0.568, −0.002).

Table B (available as a supplement to the online version of this article at

TABLE 1— Difference-in-Differences Regression Results for the Effects of Gestational Age Limit Abortion Laws on Severe Maternal Morbidity (SMM) Rate: Health Care Cost and Utilization Project Fast Stats, United States, 2010–2022

	Model 1: Any Gestational Age Limit	Model 2: Gestational Age Limit, Wk
Outcome variable: SMM rate per 10 000 in-hospital deliveries, b (95% CI)	7.673 (1.550, 13.800)	−0.282 (−0.568, 0.003)
Observations, no.	593	593
R^2	0.776	0.775
Mean of dependent variable	73.41	73.41

Note. CI = confidence interval. n = 593 state-year hospitalizations. All regressions controlled for time-varying state covariates (unemployment rate and percentage of population that is female, White, aged 18–30 y, aged 31–50 y, and aged ≥ 51 y), state fixed effects, and year fixed effects. Robust SEs were clustered at the state level. For states that had more than 1 change in gestational age limit laws during our study period, model 1 considered the earliest date that any gestational age law was implemented to be the start year of the law. For model 2, if a state changed the specific gestational age at which abortion was prohibited during our study period, we adjusted the treatment variable accordingly after the change was implemented. For example, Georgia had a gestational age limit during our entire study period, so for model 1, we coded the binary "any gestational age limit" as 1 for the entire study period. However, Georgia changed the specific week at which abortion was prohibited twice during our study period, so for model 2, we coded the "gestational age limit weeks" variable as 29 for 2010–2012, as 23 for 2013–2017, and as 20 for 2017–2022.

http://www.ajph.org) presents heterogeneity analyses for different subgroups available in HCUP Fast Stats. The association between any gestational age limits and SMM was driven by older mothers aged 35 to 55 years, who had an increase of 30.73 SMM instances per 10 000 deliveries, which was a 27.46% increase over baseline levels; mothers in the lowest income quartile (14.33, or 17.15%, increase); those whose expected payer was Medicaid or Medicare (9.68, or 6.8%, increase); and safety net hospitals (11.82, or 12.02%, increase).

Next, we conducted several sensitivity analyses and robustness checks. Table C (available as a supplement to the online version of this article at http://www.ajph.org) shows that our results were relatively unaffected by the exclusion of post–COVID-19 pandemic data, as well as post-*Dobbs* data. To further show the potential role of the *Dobbs* decision, Table D (available as a supplement to the online version of this article at http://www.ajph.org) presents several regressions in which we dropped states that changed their laws in response to the *Dobbs* decision. Our substantive results were similar in almost all these sensitivity analyses, but the coefficients increased in magnitude when we dropped states that implemented strict restrictions in response to the *Dobbs* decision.

Another concern for identification could be if states' population dynamics varied with abortion laws. Table E (available as a supplement to the online version of this article at http://www.ajph.org) shows that our results were relatively unaffected by including population control variables, as well as population-weighted regressions, which lessens this concern. Table F (available as a supplement to the online version of this article at http://www.ajph.org) shows that abortion laws were not meaningfully associated with state demographic characteristics, such as percentage Black population, percentage Hispanic population, and poverty rate.

Finally, for our second specification, we explored potential nonlinearities in the relationship between the specific week at which abortion is banned and SMM rates by using the logged and squared versions of these variables; we continued to find a negative association between more lenient laws and SMM rates (Table G, available as a supplement to the online version of this article at http://www.ajph.org).

DISCUSSION

In this nationwide quasi-experimental study, we found that restricting abortion on the basis of gestational age was associated with increased SMM rates, particularly among older patients, those whose hospitalizations were publicly funded, those served by safety net hospitals, and those living in low-income communities. Our results imply that gestational age limits were responsible for 2967 additional SMM hospitalizations in 2021 (Appendix C, available as a supplement to the online version of this article at http://www.ajph.org). This study adds to the growing literature on the public health effects of abortion laws, which consistently finds that abortion restrictions are associated with adverse health[3–6] and economic[7] consequences.

We acknowledge the limitations of this study. HCUP's SMM data are restricted to in-hospital births and patients treated in community hospitals, and data were unavailable for Idaho, Alabama, and New Hampshire. HCUP data were available only through 2022, so we could not study the impact of stricter post-*Dobbs* restrictions. Moreover, HCUP Fast Stats provides only aggregate state-level data, so we could not control for patient-level risk factors. Finally, our estimates may be biased upward if higher socioeconomic status and healthier women in restrictive states travel out of state or move to a different state to obtain abortions.

PUBLIC HEALTH IMPLICATIONS

Our results highlight the adverse public health consequences of abortion restrictions. SMM imposes negative health and economic consequences on mothers and their children and costs more than $32 billion per year through health care and ongoing complication expenses.[11] Abortion-restrictive laws that increase SMM therefore exacerbate these harms. Our findings suggest that increasing access to abortion may be an effective way to reduce SMM, particularly for women at high risk and in vulnerable situations.[12] AJPH

ABOUT THE AUTHORS

Nicole Siegal is a postdoctoral fellow at the O'Neill School of Public and Environmental Affairs, Indiana University, Bloomington. Aparna Soni is an associate professor in the Department of Health Policy & Management, Fairbanks School of Public Health, Indiana University, Indianapolis.

CORRESPONDENCE

Correspondence should be sent to Nicole Siegal, PhD, O'Neill School of Public and Environmental Affairs, Indiana University, 1315 East 10th St, Room 358, Bloomington, IN 47405 (email: nsiegal@iu.edu). Reprints can be ordered at https://www.ajph.org by clicking the "Reprints" link.

PUBLICATION INFORMATION

Full Citation: Siegal N, Soni A. The association between state gestational age limit abortion laws and severe maternal morbidity: United States, 2010–2022. *Am J Public Health*. 2026;116(3): 341–344.

Acceptance Date: September 7, 2025.

DOI: https://doi.org/10.2105/AJPH.2025.308291

ORCID iDs:
Nicole Siegal https://orcid.org/0000-0003-3220-1993

Aparna Soni https://orcid.org/0000-0003-0737-485X

CONTRIBUTORS

N. Siegal conducted the data analysis. Both authors conceptualized and designed the work, acquired and interpreted the data, drafted and edited the article, and gave final approval for publication.

ACKNOWLEDGMENTS

The efforts of coinvestigator N. Siegal were supported through the Leadership Education in Adolescent Health Program at Indiana University School of Medicine Division of Adolescent Medicine through the Health Resources and Services Administration (grant 5 T71MC45699-02-00).

We thank Guttmacher Institute for providing the information on longitudinal abortion laws across US states.

Note. The views expressed in this article are those of the authors and do not reflect the views of funders.

CONFLICTS OF INTEREST

The authors have no conflicts of interest to disclose.

HUMAN PARTICIPANT PROTECTION

No protocol approval was necessary because no human participants were involved in this study, as only de-identified and aggregated secondary data were used.

REFERENCES

1. American College of Obstetricians and Gynecologists. Periviable birth. October 2017. Available at: https://www.acog.org/-/media/project/acog/acogorg/clinical/files/obstetric-care-consensus/articles/2017/10/periviable-birth.pdf. Accessed October 8, 2025.
2. Guttmacher Institute. Abortion in the United States. April 2025. Available at: https://www.guttmacher.org/fact-sheet/induced-abortion-united-states?gad_source=1&gclid=Cj0KCQjw05i4BhDiARIsAB_2wfCkbwqijBBp6H_PZz-piU2Ry4t0G-lpoDLG39gP0aalv9AyshjAE2gaAvv7EALw_wcB. Accessed October 8, 2025.
3. Jones BS, Weitz TA. Legal barriers to second-trimester abortion provision and public health consequences. *Am J Public Health.* 2009;99(4):623–630. https://doi.org/10.2105/ajph.2007.127530
4. Karletsos D, Stoecker C, Vilda D, Theall KP, Wallace ME. Association of state gestational age limit abortion laws with infant mortality. *Am J Prev Med.* 2021;61(6):787–794. https://doi.org/10.1016/j.amepre.2021.05.022
5. Hawkins SS, Ghiani M, Harper S, Baum CF, Kaufman JS. Impact of state-level changes on maternal mortality: a population-based, quasi-experimental study. *Am J Prev Med.* 2020;58(2):165–174. https://doi.org/10.1016/j.amepre.2019.09.012
6. Pabayo R, Ehntholt A, Cook DM, Reynolds M, Muennig P, Liu SY. Laws restricting access to abortion services and infant mortality risk in the United States. *Int J Environ Res Public Health.* 2020;17(11):3773. https://doi.org/10.3390/ijerph17113773
7. Miller S, Wherry L, Foster DG. The economic consequences of being denied an abortion. National Bureau of Economic Research working paper 26662. January 2020. Available at: https://www.nber.org/papers/w26662. Accessed October 8, 2025.
8. Lindo JM, Myers CK, Schlosser A, Cunningham S. How far is too far? New evidence on abortion clinic closures, access, and abortions. *J Hum Resour.* 2020;55(4):1137–1160. https://doi.org/10.3368/jhr.55.4.1217-9254r3
9. Lindo JM, Pineda-Torres M. New evidence on the effects of mandatory waiting periods for abortion. *J Health Econ.* 2021;80:102533. https://doi.org/10.1016/j.jhealeco.2021.102533
10. Fischer S, Royer H, White C. The impacts of reduced access to abortion and family planning services on abortion, births, and contraceptive purchases. National Bureau of Economic Research working paper 23634. July 2017. Available at: https://www.nber.org/papers/w23634. Accessed October 8, 2025.
11. O'Neil SS, Platt I, Vohra D, et al. Societal cost of nine selected maternal morbidities in the United States. *PLoS ONE.* 2022;17(10):e0275656. https://doi.org/10.1371/journal.pone.0275656
12. Fink DA, Kilday D, Cao Z, et al. Trends in maternal mortality and severe maternal morbidity during delivery-related hospitalizations in the United States, 2008 to 2021. *JAMA Netw Open.* 2023;6(6):e2317641. https://doi.org/10.1001/jamanetworkopen.2023.17641

Changes in Frequency and Health of Live Births Following State Abortion Bans

Maeve E. Wallace, PhD, MPH, Yin Wang, PhD, and Charles Stoecker, PhD

See also Abortion and Public Health Impact in Post-*Dobbs* Era, pp. 321–367.

Objectives. To quantify the impact of state abortion bans on trends in fertility and preterm birth following the June 2022 US Supreme Court decision in *Dobbs v Jackson Women's Health Organization*.

Methods. We tested for changes in birth rates and preterm birth rates occurring in the first 18 months following the *Dobbs* decision by fitting 2-way fixed effects and staggered difference-in-difference models to compare trends in states that banned abortion and those that did not.

Results. We detected a statistically significant increase in the birth rate and preterm birth rate among non-Hispanic (NH) Black women above what would be expected in the absence of a ban, averaging a 3.5% increase in the birth rate and 2.1% higher incidence of preterm birth. Impacts were similar in analyses limited to births to women with Medicaid coverage, where trends among NH Black women in states that banned abortion were significantly elevated.

Conclusions. The emerging impact of state laws that ban abortion has been uneven, with trends in birth rates and preterm birth increasing especially among NH Black women in states that banned abortion. (*Am J Public Health*. 2026;116(3):345–350. https://doi.org/10.2105/AJPH.2025.308355)

AJPH March 2026, Vol. 116, No. 3

The American College of Obstetricians and Gynecologists,[1] the United Nations,[2] and the World Health Organization[3] define abortion as a necessary component of comprehensive health care and call for the removal of legal, political, and other barriers to accessing abortion care. Despite these long-standing endorsements, the increasing politicization of abortion in the United States came to a head on June 24, 2022, when the US Supreme Court decision in *Dobbs v Jackson Women's Health Organization* upheld a Mississippi law prohibiting abortion after a 15-week gestation.[4] With this decision, the court overturned *Roe v Wade*, ending the federal constitutional right to abortion and nearly 50 years of precedent. In the days and months that followed, previously unconstitutional pre-viability abortion bans went into effect in many states. As of this writing, 12 states have a total abortion ban in place, prohibiting the procedure outright with no or limited exceptions.[5]

People unable to access abortion have no choice but to continue a pregnancy to its end, most commonly in a live birth. In places where abortion is illegal, increases in the fertility rate (count of births per females of reproductive age) may therefore reflect the forced continuation of pregnancies to live births that would not have otherwise occurred had abortion been accessible.[6] This may be especially true among abortion-seeking people unable to overcome the financial, logistical, and other legal barriers to traveling for out-of-state care, receiving telemedicine, or pursuing self-managed medication abortion, options that have increased in light of the *Dobbs* decision.[7,8]

Some pieces of emergent evidence have begun to confirm this hypothesis. Bell et al.[9] reported a 1.7% increase in the fertility rate above expectation in states that implemented a ban at 6-week gestation or a total ban. They found that the increase was greater among racially minoritized people and especially among lower-income people on Medicaid.[9] Dench et al.[10] reported a 2.3% increase in births following post-*Dobbs* abortion bans relative to a synthetic control group where no ban was enforced. In older work, 2 studies of the 6-week abortion ban imposed by the state of Texas in 2021 found it was associated with an increase in the count[6] and rate[11] of live births occurring in the months and years following the policy.

To date, there are few empirical studies of changes to trends in maternal and infant health outcomes and inequities following post-*Dobbs* state abortion bans. Preliminary evidence detects an increase in infant mortality in states banning abortion,[12,13] most notably among births to Black women,[12] confirming prior work associating pre-*Dobbs* state abortion regulations with increases in infant mortality.[14–16] No studies to date have identified associations between post-*Dobbs* abortion bans and trends in preterm birth, a leading cause of infant mortality and an adverse birth outcome marked by long-standing racial and economic inequities and a troubling shift in severity in recent years.[17]

Researchers posit that in the United States, centuries of racial, gender, and economic oppression have restricted access to institutional power and resources among racialized minorities and low-income women, rendering them least able to obtain a timely and safe abortion (i.e., least able to exercise bodily autonomy) in a highly restrictive environment.[18] These circumstances are preceded by racial inequities in access to contraception and are followed by deeply entrenched inequities in maternal and infant health, including preterm birth and maternal and infant mortality.[19]

The purpose of this study was to analyze the first full year of national birth data following the federal constitutional reversal of abortion rights. This work enhances earlier evidence that relied on provisional data and a modeling approach that requires more assumptions in support of causal inference. We applied a rigorous difference-in-difference approach to evaluate the extent to which state abortion bans implemented following the *Dobbs* decision led to changes in the frequency and health of infants born in states that banned abortion. We hypothesized that within states that banned abortion, Black and low-income women—those with limited access to institutional power and resources—would be especially affected, amplifying already vast inequities in reproductive health.

METHODS

We analyzed birth records in the restricted use natality files maintained by the National Center for Health Statistics for the period June 2021 through December 2023. From these data, we ascertained information about maternal state of residence, maternal race and ethnicity, type of health insurance, and gestational weeks at birth. We obtained the monthly count of births by state for the total population and to non-Hispanic (NH) Black women. We restricted the sample to births covered by Medicaid as an indicator of limited economic resources and extracted monthly count of births again for the total population, and among NH White and NH Black women separately.

We identified preterm births as those occurring before 37 weeks of gestation and obtained the monthly count of preterm births among the total population and among births covered by Medicaid, among those to NH Black women, and finally among those to NH Black women enrolled in Medicaid.

For the purposes of estimating trends in birth rates and preterm birth rates per 100 000, we used data on the total population of females aged 15 to 44 years in each state (NH Black females aged 15–44 years in race-stratified models) as the rate denominator. We obtained these data from the State Population by Characteristics provided by the US Census Bureau.[20] We used a denominator of reproductive aged women (females aged 15–44 years) for our evaluation of preterm birth rates to avoid selection bias introduced by a live births denominator. It is possible that the *Dobbs* decision and the rapidly changing abortion policy climate that followed resulted in fundamental changes in who selects into fertility after the *Dobbs* decision, thereby changing the composition of pregnancies continuing to live births in ways that may affect population-level trends in preterm birth.

Exposure

The exposure under study was a total abortion ban implemented immediately following the *Dobbs* decision. This included 12 states (AL, AR, ID, KY, LA, MS, MO, OK, SD, TN, TX, and WV) that imposed bans between June 24, 2022, and August 25, 2022. We excluded Indiana because it implemented an abortion ban later in 2023, only 4 months before the end of our study period. We additionally excluded North Dakota and Wisconsin because there was considerable debate in the months and year following the *Dobbs* decision over the legality of abortion in these states where there were bans enforced and blocked or overturned, causing confusion for patients and providers and making their treatment status difficult to quantify.

Statistical Analysis

We used a difference-in-difference design that compared changes in birth rates between states with abortion bans (treated group) and those without abortion bans (control group) before and after the enforcement of a total abortion ban following the *Dobbs* decision in June 2022. We fit Poisson models with a population denominator offset (females of reproductive age) to estimate relative changes in birth rates and preterm birth rates associated with the bans. The models controlled for state-fixed effects, year-by-month fixed effects, and state-level covariates, including the annual unemployment rate, percentage of the population with a bachelor's degree or higher, median household income (logarithmic form), poverty rate, percentage of the population with no health insurance coverage, and percentage of the population that is NH Black, NH White, and Hispanic. Covariate measures were derived from the American Community Survey.[21] Standard errors were clustered at the state level to address the serial correlation in birth rates within a state.

In addition to modeling trends in the total population, we fit models restricted to births covered by Medicaid and to births to NH Black women (as well as among persons who were both Black and on Medicaid) to assess the degree to which state abortion bans may contribute to racial and economic inequities in access to abortion and preterm birth.

Five of the 12 state bans under study went into effect on the date of the *Dobbs* decision (June 24, 2022); the other 7 bans took place up to 3 months later. To account for this, we also implemented staggered treatment timing differences-in-differences approaches using the month each state's ban went into effect as the start of the state's treatment period. We implemented this approach using a 2-way fixed effects estimator as well as the staggered differences-in-differences estimators proposed by Sun and Abraham,[22] de Chaisemartin and D'Haultfœuille,[23] and Butts and Gardner.[24]

We also estimated event-study models to assess whether the outcomes followed parallel trends in the preintervention period and to investigate the dynamic impacts of the *Dobbs* decision on birth outcomes over time across the postintervention period.

RESULTS

Descriptive distributions of births stratified by policy exposure (states that implemented an abortion ban and those that did not) are contained in Appendix Table A (available as a supplement to the online version of this article at http://www.ajph.org).

Differences in birth rates between states that implemented bans and those that did not, relative to the month before the *Dobbs* decision, are shown in Figure 1. The differences between treated and control states are similar in the pre- and postperiods for the total population (Figure 1a), indicating nonparallel pretrends. For NH Black births (Figure 1b), the 95% confidence interval (CI) includes zero in 8 of 11 preperiod estimates, but only 2 of 19 postperiod estimates. Estimates and CIs depicted in Figure 1 can be found in Appendix Table B.

In the final, fully adjusted difference-in-difference models, the monthly total birth rates in states with abortion bans increased by 2% over the first 18 months following the *Dobbs* decision, compared with what would be expected in the absence of the ban (incident rate ratio = 1.020; 95% CI = 1.009, 1.031; $P < .001$; Table 1). However, this estimate should be interpreted with caution given the substantial evidence of a nonparallel pretrend in the total group. Furthermore, among NH Black women where there is less evidence of nonparallel pretrends, point estimates became notably larger in the post-*Dobbs* period, indicating an increase of 3.5% in birth rates (incident rate ratio = 1.035; 95% CI = 1.020, 1.050; $P < .001$; Table 1).

These findings were similar in models restricted to births covered by Medicaid (Table 1). Point estimates for the association between abortion bans and increased birth rates among Medicaid participants were higher than in the total population, but overlapping CIs indicate a lack of precision. Event-studies birth rates among Medicaid participants and NH Black Medicaid participants are shown in Appendix Figures A and B, respectively.

The suggestion of uneven impact was mirrored in the analysis of preterm birth rates following the *Dobbs* decision (Table 2). We estimated a 2% increase in preterm birth rates among NH Black women associated with the bans (incident rate ratio = 1.021; 95% CI = 1.001, 1.041; $P < .05$), and smaller increases that were not statistically significant in the total population. Estimates of the impact on preterm birth rates generally showed limited evidence of nonparallel pretrends (Appendix Figures C–F).

Results from the supplemental analyses that applied a staggered treatment differences-in-differences approach are shown in Appendix Tables C and D and Figures G through N. Similar to the primary analysis, these models estimated postban changes in birth rates of 2.1% to 4.2% (Appendix Table C). Changes in preterm birth rates were highest among NH Black women, but these estimates are imprecise and not statistically significant (Appendix Table D).

AJPH March 2026, Vol. 116, No. 3

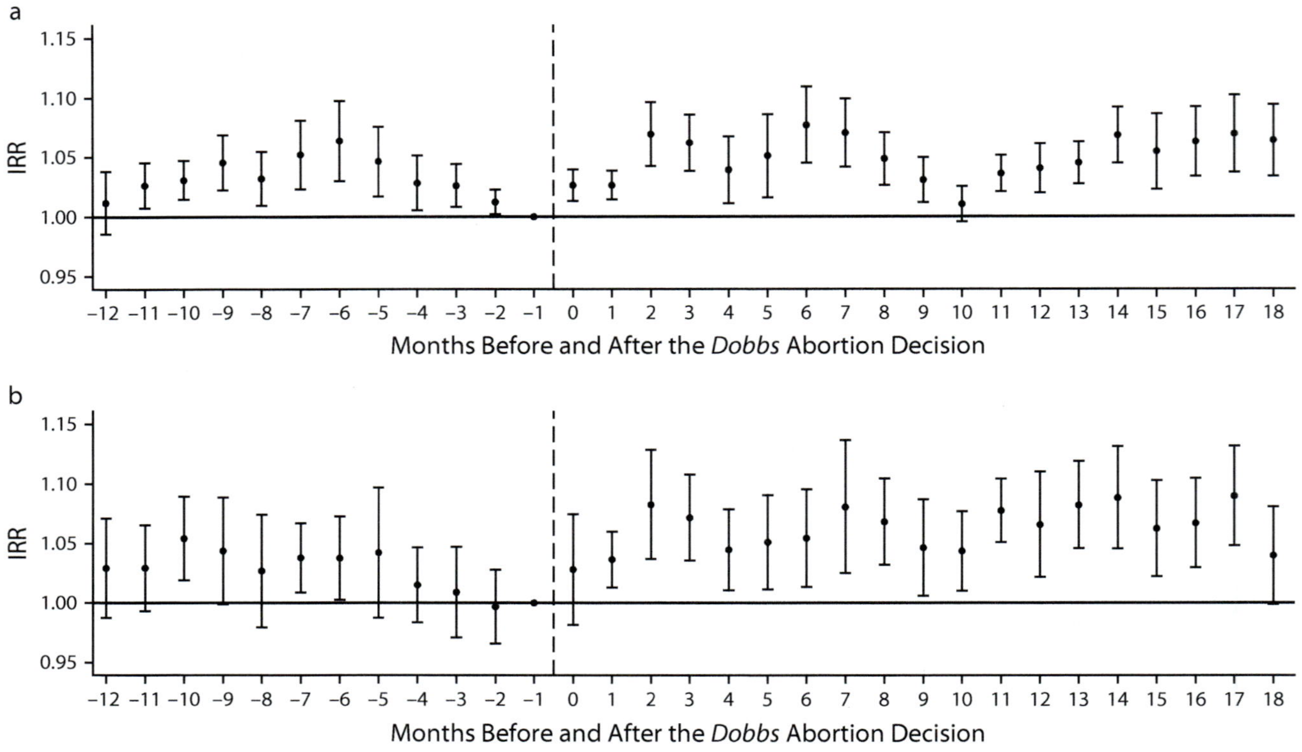

FIGURE 1— Event Study of Associations Between Announcement of *Dobbs* Decision and Birth Rates in (a) the Total Population and (b) Among Non-Hispanic Black Women: United States, June 2021–December 2023

Note. IRR = incidence rate ratio.

DISCUSSION

In this analysis of the first 18 months of births occurring since the US Supreme Court overturned the federal constitutional right to abortion care in *Dobbs v Jackson Women's Health Organization*, our study supports earlier evidence of the impact of subsequent state abortion bans on fertility and infant health. Our most salient finding is the indication of an uneven impact of state abortion bans and their potential contribution to worsening inequities in reproductive health in the United States. Although our estimate of an increase in birth rates in the total population violates the nonparallel pretrends assumption, among NH Black women, the case is clearer. Birth rates and incidence of preterm birth increased significantly among NH Black women in states that banned abortion. These findings suggest that at least some of these births may have been to women who were unable to access a wanted abortion and had no choice but to continue the pregnancy to birth. The factors related to their inability to overcome an abortion ban—limited institutional power, financial and social

TABLE 1— Associations Between Announcement of *Dobbs* Decision and Birth Rates, by Race and Medicaid Enrollment Status: United States, June 2021–December 2023

	Percent Change	IRR (95% CI)
Total births		
All races	0.020	1.02 (1.01, 1.03)
Non-Hispanic Black	0.035	1.04 (1.02, 1.05)
Births among Medicaid participants		
All races	0.030	1.03 (1.01, 1.05)
Non-Hispanic Black	0.420	1.04 (1.02, 1.06)

Note. CI = confidence interval; IRR = incidence rate ratio. Treated states included AL, AR, ID, KY, LA, MS, MO, OK, SD, TN, TX, and WV. All models included 1488 state-month observations. Estimates were derived from a covariate-adjusted Poisson regression model that used log birth count as outcome and log female population aged 15 to 44 years as denominator offset. The incidence rate ratio represents the birth rate ratio between the post- and pretreatment periods. Percent change was obtained by the incidence rate ratio minus 1.

TABLE 2— Associations Between Announcement of *Dobbs* Decision and Preterm Birth Rates, by Race and Medicaid Enrollment Status: United States, June 2021–December 2023

	Percent Change	IRR (95% CI)
Total preterm births		
All races	0.015	1.02 (0.996, 1.035)
Non-Hispanic Black	0.021	1.02 (1.001, 1.041)
Preterm births among Medicaid participants		
All races	0.012	1.01 (0.99, 1.03)
Non-Hispanic Black	0.022	1.02 (0.99, 1.06)

Note. CI = confidence interval; IRR = incidence rate ratio. Treated states included AL, AR, ID, KY, LA, MS, MO, OK, SD, TN, TX, and WV. All models included 1488 state-month observations. Estimates were derived from a covariate-adjusted Poisson regression model that used log birth count as outcome and log female population aged 15 to 44 years as denominator offset. The incidence rate ratio represents the birth rate ratio between the post- and pre treatment periods. Percent change was obtained by the incidence rate ratio minus 1.

resources—may subsequently increase their likelihood of experiencing a preterm birth. States that implemented abortion bans after the *Dobbs* decision are those with the largest proportion of Black residents; therefore, not only may NH Black women be most affected by a ban, they are most likely to be exposed to it. As a result, such policies may be identified as substantial contributors to the widening of racial health inequities in the coming years.[25]

We did not find evidence of a unique impact of economic position alone, with estimates among the Medicaid population similar to that of the total population, albeit imprecise. Rather, the intersection of racial and economic oppression was evident where the magnitude of the point estimates for trends in total birth rates and preterm birth rates were highest among NH Black women with Medicaid coverage.

Our findings are consistent with prior work that found a 2% increase in births to NH Black women with a modeling approach that relaxed the parallel trends assumption in the preperiod using Bayesian techniques,[9] a second work that found a 2.3% increase in fertility that used a synthetic differences-in-differences technique to satisfy the parallel trends assumption,[10] and a third work that found a 3.2% increase in births to Black women in counties where the state abortion ban increased the distance to care to more than 300 miles.[26] Our analysis contributes to this small but growing body of evidence by providing another estimate of the population health consequences associated with abortion bans.

This study has important limitations to consider. First, state abortion bans were not randomly assigned, and important differences in the legal and geographic access to abortion between states may be at play. Second, several of the samples analyzed here display nonparallel pretrends. Even the most comparable groups (births to NH Black women in treatment and control states) exhibit some small pretreatment differences. Third, we rely on administrative birth data—vital records—which lack circumstantial details about pregnancy desirability or unfulfilled attempts to access abortion care. Fourth, we lacked statistical power to further stratify models by state and month for smaller groups that may have less ability to overcome barriers to reproductive health care and experience inequities in preterm birth (e.g., American Indian people or immigrant groups).

This analysis suggests that state abortion bans are having an emerging impact on population health, with evidence of an increasing incidence of birth and preterm births, most robustly among NH Black women. *AJPH*

ABOUT THE AUTHORS

Maeve E. Wallace is with the Mel and Enid Zuckerman College of Public Health, University of Arizona, Tucson. At the time of this study, Yin Wang and Charles Stoecker were with the Celia Scott Weatherhead School of Public Health and Tropical Medicine, Tulane University, New Orleans, LA.

CORRESPONDENCE

Correspondence should be sent to Maeve E. Wallace, Department of Health Promotion Sciences, Mel and Enid Zuckerman College of Public Health, University of Arizona, 1295 N Martin Ave, Tucson, AZ 85719 (e-mail: maevewallace@arizona.edu). Reprints can be ordered at https://www.ajph.org by clicking the "Reprints" link.

PUBLICATION INFORMATION

Full Citation: Wallace ME, Wang Y, Stoecker C. Changes in frequency and health of live births following state abortion bans. *Am J Public Health*. 2026;116(3):345–350.

Acceptance Date: November 9, 2025.

DOI: https://doi.org/10.2105/AJPH.2025.308355

ORCID iDs:

Yin Wang https://orcid.org/0000-0002-3554-656X

Charles Stoecker https://orcid.org/0000-0001-5438-9312

CONTRIBUTORS

M. E. Wallace and C. Stoecker conceptualized the research question and designed the study. M. E. Wallace and Y. Wang acquired the data. Y. Wang conducted the analysis. All authors interpreted the analytic findings, drafted and critically revised the manuscript, and approved the final version for publication.

ACKNOWLEDGMENTS

Research reported in this article was supported by the Eunice Kennedy Shriver National Institute of Child Health & Human Development of the National Institutes of Health (award no. R01HD096070).

Note. The contents are solely the responsibility of the authors and do not necessarily represent the official views of the National Institutes of Health.

CONFLICTS OF INTEREST

The authors have no conflicts of interest to report.

HUMAN PARTICIPANT PROTECTION

This analysis of de-identified, secondary data was deemed not human subjects research by the University of Arizona institutional review board.

REFERENCES

1. American College of Obstetrics and Gynecologists, Gynecologists' Committee on Health Care for Underserved Women, Gynecologists' Abortion Access, Training Expert Work Group. Increasing access to abortion: ACOG committee opinion, number 815. *Obstet Gynecol.* 2020;136(6):e107–e115. https://doi.org/10.1097/AOG.0000000000004176
2. United Nations Dept of Economic and Social Affairs Population Division. Abortion policies and reproductive health around the world. 2014. Available at: https://www.un.org/en/development/desa/population/publications/pdf/policy/AbortionPoliciesReproductiveHealth.pdf. Accessed December 10, 2025.
3. World Health Organization. Maternal mortality: fact sheet: to improve maternal health, barriers that limit access to quality maternal health services must be identified and addressed at all levels of the health system. 2014. Available at: https://apps.who.int/iris/handle/10665/112318. Accessed October 10, 2020.
4. *Dobbs v Jackson Women's Health Organization*, 597 US 215 (2022).
5. Kaiser Family Foundation. Abortion in the United States Dashboard. 2025. Available at: https://www.kff.org/womens-health-policy/dashboard/abortion-in-the-u-s-dashboard. Accessed February 18, 2025.
6. Bell SO, Stuart EA, Gemmill A. Texas' 2021 ban on abortion in early pregnancy and changes in live births. *JAMA.* 2023;330(3):281–282. https://doi.org/10.1001/jama.2023.12034
7. Aiken ARA, Wells ES, Gomperts R, Scott JG. Provision of medications for self-managed abortion before and after the *Dobbs v Jackson Women's Health Organization* decision. *JAMA.* 2024;331(18):1558–1564. https://doi.org/10.1001/jama.2024.4266
8. Fuerst M, Mandelbaum A, Nacev E, Rodriguez M. Trends in interstate abortion travel to Oregon following the Dobbs court decision. *Contraception.* 2024;138:110520. https://doi.org/10.1016/j.contraception.2024.110520
9. Bell SO, Franks AM, Arbour D, et al. US abortion bans and fertility. *JAMA.* 2025;333(15):1324–1332. https://doi.org/10.1001/jama.2024.28527
10. Dench D, Pineda-Torres M, Myers C. The effects of post-Dobbs abortion bans on fertility. *J Public Econ.* 2024;234:105124. https://doi.org/10.1016/j.jpubeco.2024.105124
11. Caraher D. Do abortion bans affect reproductive and infant health? Evidence from Texas's 2021 ban and its impact on health disparities. 2024. Available at: https://papers.ssrn.com/sol3/papers.cfm?abstract_id=4911886. Accessed February 18, 2025.
12. Gemmill A, Franks AM, Anjur-Dietrich S, et al. US abortion bans and infant mortality. *JAMA.* 2025;333(15):1315–1323. https://doi.org/10.1001/jama.2024.28517
13. Singh P, Gallo MF. National trends in infant mortality in the US After Dobbs. *JAMA Pediatr.* 2024;178(12):1364–1366. https://doi.org/10.1001/jamapediatrics.2024.4276
14. Gemmill A, Margerison CE, Stuart EA, Bell SO. Infant deaths after Texas' 2021 ban on abortion in early pregnancy. *JAMA Pediatr.* 2024;178(8):784–791. https://doi.org/10.1001/jamapediatrics.2024.0885
15. Karletsos D, Stoecker C, Vilda D, Theall KP, Wallace ME. Association of state gestational age limit abortion laws with infant mortality. *Am J Prev Med.* 2021;61(6):787–794. https://doi.org/10.1016/j.amepre.2021.05.022
16. Pabayo R, Ehntholt A, Cook DM, Reynolds M, Muennig P, Liu SY. Laws restricting access to abortion services and infant mortality risk in the United States. *Int J Environ Res Public Health.* 2020;17(11):3773. https://doi.org/10.3390/ijerph17113773
17. Martin JA, Osterman MJK. Shifts in the distribution of births by gestational age: United States, 2014–2022. *Natl Vital Stat Rep.* 2024;73(1):1–11.
18. Jung C, Oviedo J, Nippita S. Abortion care in the United States—current evidence and future directions. *NEJM Evid.* 2023;2(4):EVIDra2200300. https://doi.org/10.1056/EVIDra2200300
19. Kheyfets A, Dhaurali S, Feyock P, et al. The impact of hostile abortion legislation on the United States maternal mortality crisis: a call for increased abortion education. *Front Public Health.* 2023;11:1291668. https://doi.org/10.3389/fpubh.2023.1291668
20. US Census Bureau. State population by characteristics: 2020–2024. 2024. Available at: https://www.census.gov/data/tables/time-series/demo/popest/2020s-state-detail.html. Accessed December 12, 2024.
21. US Census Bureau. American Community Survey 1-year data (2005–2023). 2024. Available at: https://www.census.gov/data/developers/data-sets/acs-1year.html. Accessed December 1, 2024.
22. Sun LY, Abraham S. Estimating dynamic treatment effects in event studies with heterogeneous treatment effects. *J Econometrics.* 2021;225(2):175–199. https://doi.org/10.1016/j.jeconom.2020.09.006
23. de Chaisemartin C, D'Haultfœuille X. Two-way fixed effects estimators with heterogeneous treatment effects. *Am Econ Rev.* 2020;110(9):2964–2996. https://doi.org/10.1257/aer.20181169
24. Butts K, Gardner J. did2s: two-stage difference-in-differences. *The R Journal.* 2022. Available at: https://journal.r-project.org/articles/RJ-2022-048. Accessed December 11, 2025.
25. Ward JB, Gartner DR, Keyes KM, Fliss MD, McClure ES, Robinson WR. How do we assess a racial disparity in health? Distribution, interaction, and interpretation in epidemiological studies. *Ann Epidemiol.* 2019;29:1–7. https://doi.org/10.1016/j.annepidem.2018.09.007
26. Myers C, Dench DL, Pineda-Torres M. The road not taken: how driving distance and appointment availability shape the effects of abortion bans. National Bureau of Economic Research Working Paper 33548. 2025. Available at: https://www.nber.org/system/files/working_papers/w33548/w33548.pdf. Accessed March 18, 2025.

Examining Post-*Dobbs* Changes in Abortion Use at 3 Southern Michigan Clinics, July 2021–June 2023

Mikaela H. Smith, PhD, Caroline Sucher, BS, Alison Norris, MD, PhD, Vanessa K. Dalton, MD, MPH, and Sarah D. Compton, PhD, MPH

See also Abortion and Public Health Impact in Post-*Dobbs* Era, pp. 321–367.

Objectives. To examine changes in abortion service delivery for the years before (July 2021–June 2022) and after *Dobbs v Jackson Women's Health* (July 2022–June 2023) at 3 Planned Parenthood clinics in southern Michigan, when several states enacted laws further restricting abortion access, and Michigan became a destination for individuals in restrictive states.

Methods. We used monthly abortion data from 3 Michigan clinics to calculate the mean number of monthly abortions and changes in proportions for gestation, method, and patient state of residence for the 2 time periods.

Results. Mean monthly abortions increased from 358 before *Dobbs* to 575 after *Dobbs*. Simultaneously, out-of-state patients increased from 383 before *Dobbs* to 1145 after *Dobbs* and received a larger share of total abortions. Methods shifted slightly, with medication abortions decreasing from 58% to 53% and procedural abortions at less than 14 weeks increasing from 31% to 36%. Most out-of-state patients came from Indiana and Ohio.

Conclusions. The increasing number of out-of-state patients and increased provision of procedural abortions represent both increased need among patients from restrictive states and adaptability among providers in protective states such as Michigan—underscoring changes in care amid the rapidly evolving abortion landscape in the United States. (*Am J Public Health*. 2026;116(3):351–358. https://doi.org/10.2105/AJPH.2025.308305)

AJPH March 2026, Vol. 116, No. 3

Access to abortion, which is common, safe, and necessary reproductive health care, is constrained for many people who need abortion care. Many people live far from an abortion provider,[1,2] find the cost of an abortion not covered by health insurance to be prohibitive,[3] and live in states with laws that restrict access by limiting how care can be delivered and via gestational limits.[4] Given the wide variation of state laws, abortion access in the United States is determined in part by the state in which a pregnant person resides. Such state-level disparities have become more severe since the Supreme Court decided *Dobbs v Jackson Women's Health Organization* and struck down *Roe v Wade* and *Planned Parenthood v Casey* in June 2022. The *Dobbs* decision returned the issue of regulating abortion to individual states. As of July 2, 2025, according to KFF,[5] complete abortion bans are now law in 12 states, and an additional 6 states restrict abortion at early gestational limits (e.g., 6 weeks since last menstrual period in Florida, Georgia, Iowa, and South Carolina, and 12 weeks in North Carolina and Nebraska). Abortion is legal, with limits ranging from 18 weeks to viability in 23 states and protected (no gestational limit) in 9 states, including Michigan. State-level abortion policy continues to be a fluid situation.

Before recent legal changes, people seeking abortions in Michigan were subject to numerous regulatory barriers that had been passed by the state legislature.[6] Michigan, like other states, has both patient-level and provider-level restrictions on abortion care—some of which have been recently enjoined or repealed, and some of which remain. At the individual level, patients were required to receive state-directed counseling that included language designed to discourage abortion and then wait 24 hours after this counseling before receiving their abortion. Michigan also requires that the parent of a minor give their consent before the minor can receive their abortion. At the provider level, facilities that provide abortions must meet certain non–evidence-based requirements—unnecessary for patient safety—related to their physical structure, equipment, and staffing.

Despite these regulations, recent abortion-related legal changes[6] have also made Michigan a safe haven (i.e., a destination state amid several restrictive states) for those seeking abortion. In 2022, a ballot initiative successfully protected abortion services in Michigan; in 2023, a 1931 law that banned abortion (and had been unenforced for decades) was officially repealed; and in 2024, the 24-hour waiting period, restrictions limiting abortion provision to physicians, and several facility regulations were enjoined as incompatible with the 2022 change to the state constitution.[7] Publicly available data from the Society of Family Planning's #WeCount project show that monthly abortions in Michigan rose from 2610 in April 2022 to 3260 in December 2024—a 25% increase.[8] Given the uncertainty of abortion legality in its nearby states, Michigan will remain an important site of abortion care.

Even before the recent changes to Michigan's abortion laws, the state was a destination for abortion care for residents of more restrictive states surrounding it—particularly Ohio and Indiana. In the year following the *Dobbs* decision, both Ohio and Indiana either passed or enacted restrictive abortion laws, creating confusion and reducing availability of abortion in those states.[7,9] In August 2023, Indiana enacted a total abortion ban,[10] which may increase the number of people seeking abortion care coming to Michigan or other haven states, such as Illinois or Pennsylvania, in the future. Meanwhile, in Michigan, many providers of abortion services have added capacity to their clinics to better absorb increased demand for abortion.[11,12] The Guttmacher Institute's Monthly Abortion Provision Study compared data from 2020 to 2023 and documented a greater than 50% increase in the number of patients coming into Michigan from out of state, with patients in 2023 coming from Ohio, Indiana, and Texas.[13]

While these publicly available sources capture total number of abortions, they are not able to capture more disaggregated data such as gestation at abortion, method type, and patient state of residence. A small number of state-based studies have also been conducted. A study of Ohio abortion clinics documents monthly changes in these abortion characteristics surrounding *Dobbs*; however, Ohio underwent legislative changes in the immediate aftermath of *Dobbs* that restricted access in the state.[9] Studies from 3 other abortion haven states (Illinois,[14,15] Massachusetts,[16] and Oregon[17]) found increases in abortion counts, percentage of out-of-state patients, and gestation at abortion using patient-level data.

Thus, this study serves as a useful companion analysis for a state in which abortion remained protected during this volatile time, and which was situated geographically close to more restrictive states. Investigations into abortion clinic volume in protected states after *Dobbs* have been limited. In this article, we used clinic-level data from 3 Planned Parenthood of Michigan (PPMI) clinics to describe changes in abortion in the year preceding and the year following the *Dobbs* decision. By drawing on data from the same 3 clinics during these 2 years of legal turbulence, we can observe patterns in abortion service delivery, including gestation, method, and state of residence, with more nuance.

METHODS

Data for the 3 clinics in this analysis are from an ongoing monthly survey of standalone abortion facilities in the eastern Midwest. We began data collection in 2020; the data analyzed here represent abortions that took place from July 2021 through June 2023. Each month, staff at abortion facilities compile abortion count data, including information about how many abortions were provided by method type, gestational age, and patient state of residence. Data are collected through a secure REDCap portal and stored on a secure server. Any standalone abortion facility in the region was eligible to participate; data for this analysis represent all Michigan facilities that agreed to participate during the study period. Specifically, they represent abortions from the 3 PPMI facilities that provide both procedural and medication abortion at the time of this study, most of which are located in southern Michigan. They account for approximately 10% of abortions in the state.[18] All 3 participating facilities are in the southern part of the state, making them more accessible to abortion seekers traveling from Indiana and Ohio. Facilities were compensated for participation.

We examined changes in abortion characteristics and state of patient residence before and after *Dobbs*. Specifically, we summed the monthly counts from the 3 participating PPMI facilities for each month. We then calculated the monthly mean for 2 time periods: before *Dobbs* (July 2021 through June 2022) and after *Dobbs* (July 2022 through June 2023). We also calculated, for each month and each time period, the number and proportion of abortions by gestation (< 12 weeks, 12–13 weeks, 14–17 weeks, and ≥ 18 weeks), method (procedural or medication), and patient state of residence. We also calculated the percentage of patients coming from out of state versus in state for care.

RESULTS

Our study showed an increasing number of abortions in these 3 PPMI clinics between July 2021 and June 2023 (Figure 1). Specifically, before *Dobbs*, there were 4296 abortions (monthly mean = 358); after *Dobbs*, this increased to 6901 (monthly mean = 575)—a 61% increase.

Regarding the method of abortion (medication vs procedural), there were 2501 medication abortions and 1791 procedural abortions before *Dobbs*, representing 58% and 42% of pre-*Dobbs* abortions, respectively. After *Dobbs*, there were 3650 medication abortions and 3249 procedural abortions, representing 53% and 47% of post-*Dobbs* abortions, respectively. Thus, we observed a relative increase in the number of procedural abortions, as the total number of abortions also increased.

We observed small changes in the relative number of procedural abortions taking place at less than 14 weeks gestation. Specifically, before *Dobbs*, 1327 procedural abortions (31%) were at less than 14 weeks gestation, and 464 procedural abortions (11%) were at 14 weeks or later. After *Dobbs*, this was 2476 procedural abortions (36%) at less than 14 weeks and 773 (11%) at 14 weeks or later.

In the post-*Dobbs* period, the relative number of out-of-state patients increased compared with those from Michigan (Figure 2). Before *Dobbs*, 383 abortions, representing 9% of patients, were provided to out-of-state patients. After *Dobbs*, this value was 1145, representing 17% of patients—a 199% increase. The number of Michiganders who obtained an abortion increased from 3913 before *Dobbs* (91% of abortions) to 5756 after *Dobbs* (83% of abortions)—a 47% increase.

In both time periods, most out-of-state patients receiving abortion care came from Ohio and Indiana, and there were substantial increases in the number of patients from these 2 states after *Dobbs* (Figure 3). The total number of

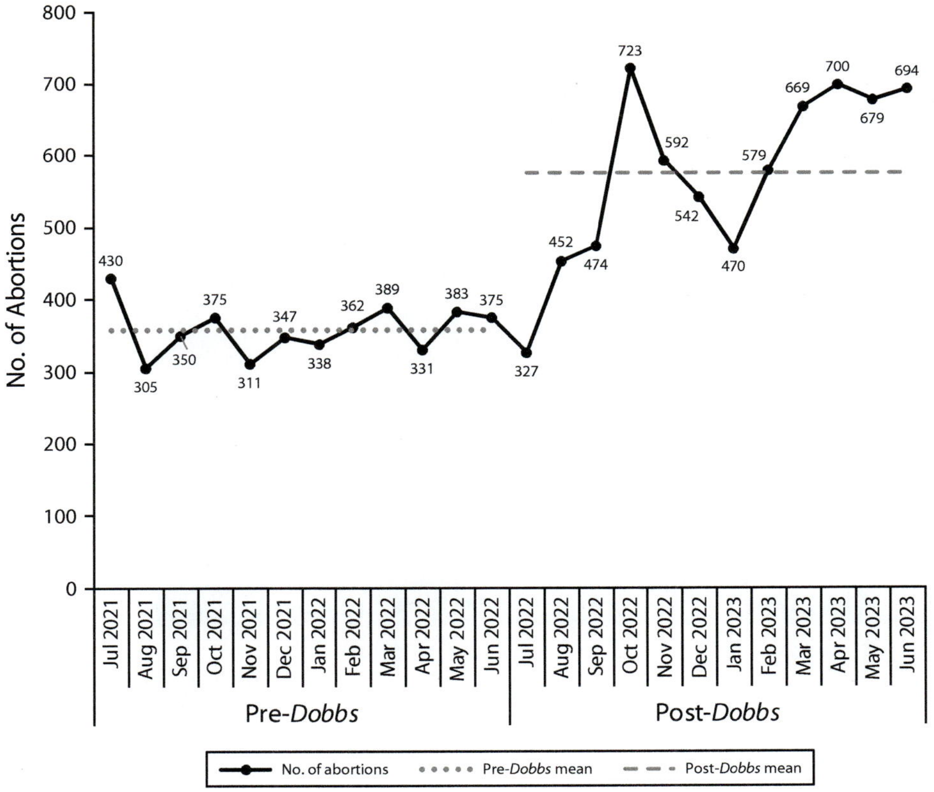

FIGURE 1— Number of Abortions by Month and Pre- and Post-*Dobbs* Means at 3 Sites in Michigan: July 2021–June 2023

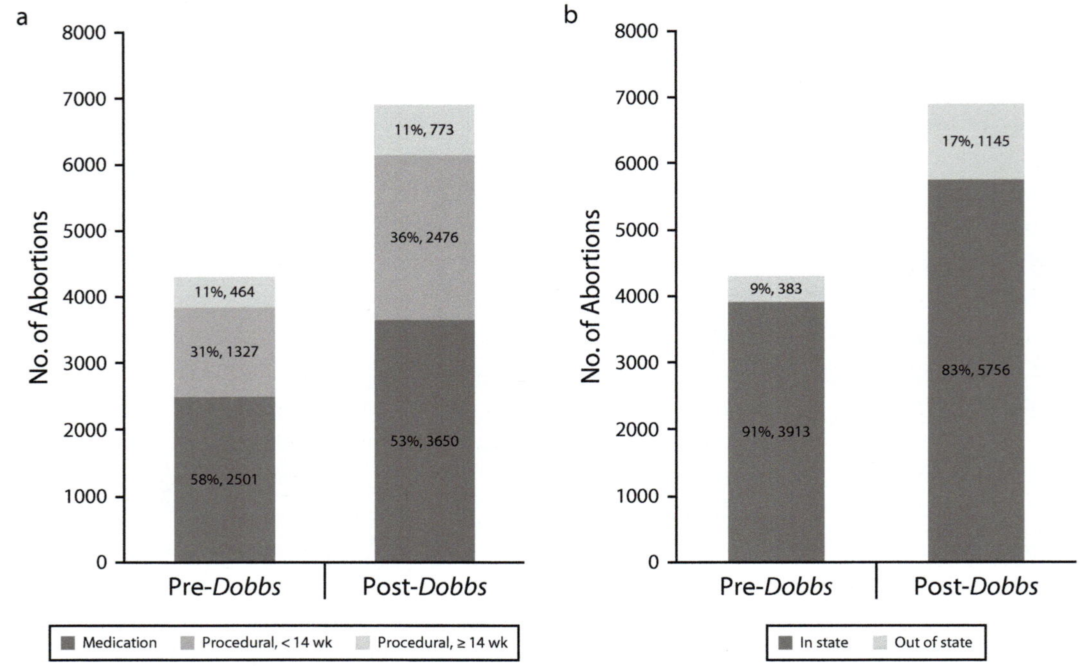

FIGURE 2— **Number and Percentage of Abortions in Michigan Before and After *Dobbs* by (a) Procedure Type and (b) Michigan Residence Status: July 2021–June 2023**

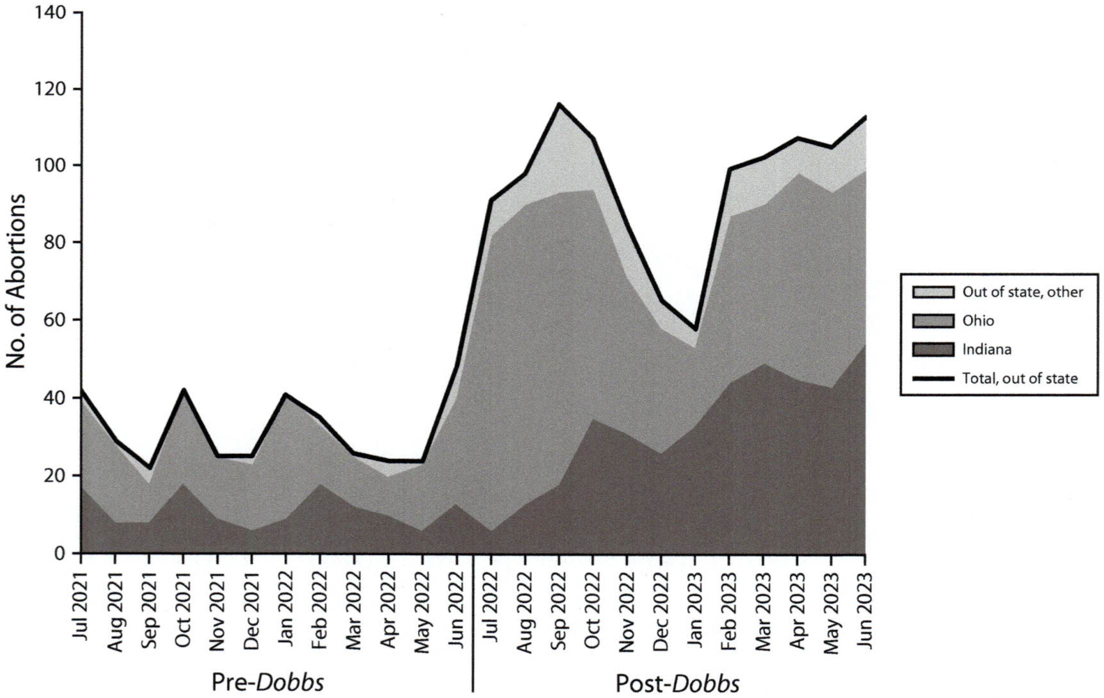

FIGURE 3— **Number and Percentage of Abortions in Michigan Among Out-of-State Patients by Month: July 2021–June 2023**

patients from Indiana increased from 134 before *Dobbs* (representing 35% of out-of-state patients) to 397 after *Dobbs* (also 35% of out-of-state patients)—a 196% increase. Similarly, the number of patients from Ohio increased from 222 before *Dobbs* (58%) to 611 after *Dobbs* (53%)—a 275% increase.

There was also an increase in the total number of states from which patients traveled for abortion care, from 17 states before *Dobbs* to 24 states in the post-*Dobbs* period (Figure 4). The new travelers were mainly from states in the South (Alabama, Georgia, South Carolina, and Oklahoma) and from Wisconsin, another midwestern state that enforced an abortion ban.

DISCUSSION

This study documents a marked increase in abortion volume at 3 PPMI clinics in southern Michigan in the year following the *Dobbs* decision. Notably, while there were more abortions among Michigan residents, there was a larger increase in people traveling from other states. A study estimating how abortion counts might increase if nearby states banned abortion suggested that Michigan would see a 21% increase in case load from out-of-state patients alone[19]; our data showed that the number of abortions among participating clinics increased 27% from out-of-state patients.

In particular, we saw many patients coming from Ohio and Indiana, which both enacted abortion restrictions for at least some portion of the months covered in this study. Specifically, Ohio had a 6-week ban in place immediately after *Dobbs* through September 14, 2022[9]; the large portion of the area representing Ohio's abortions in Figure 1 is likely a large factor in the especially high jump in total abortions we observed in the immediate aftermath of *Dobbs*. While Indiana passed a total abortion ban in September, it was in place for only a week before being blocked by the courts (it eventually went into effect in August 2023, after our study period).[7] The near–total ban Indiana currently has in place suggests that there will continue to be demand for abortion services for Indiana residents.[10] While individuals from Indiana might also be able to access services in Illinois, the location of the 3 clinics in our study, in the southern part of Michigan, allows closer access for some Indiana residents. The increase in abortion provision for these patients represents both providers increasing their availability for care and more patients traveling long distances, and paying related costs, to receive their care.

Similar increases in provision of abortion services to out-of-state residents have been seen in Illinois, Massachusetts, Ohio, and Oregon.[9,14–17] While Michigan will continue to be a haven state for abortion care given the 2022 change to the state constitution protecting abortion services, it is important to note that adding travel costs to the cost of an abortion makes the procedure unaffordable for some people. Furthermore, while Michigan's mandated 24-hour waiting period was enjoined by a state judge in June of 2024,[20] when it was in effect, it imposed additional waiting time and subsequent cost on patients, which were likely exacerbated by the increased volume of patients who were seeking services from out of state after *Dobbs*.[21]

Nationwide, there had been an increase in the number of abortions occurring in the formal health care system that started before the *Dobbs* decision, and almost all states that did not enact a ban after *Dobbs* have seen an increase in the number of abortions provided in the post-*Dobbs* period compared with 2020, the last time national estimates were available. Specifically, the #WeCount study estimates a 14% increase in the number of abortions nationally from April 2022 to December 2024.[8] Similarly, the Monthly Abortion Provision Study suggests an 11% increase in abortions from 2020 to 2023.[13] Our data from Michigan point in the same direction, even more sharply: in these 3 clinics in southern Michigan, the increase was more than 60%—from 4296 abortions in the 12 months before *Dobbs* to 6901 in the 12 months after *Dobbs*. Importantly, while there was a large increase in the number of abortions provided at these clinics, there has not been an increase in the overall abortion rate in Michigan, where it was 15.0 per 100 000 in 2021, 14.5 per 100 000 in 2022, and 15.0 per 100 000 in 2023.[22]

Clinic- and state-level changes are likely related to our findings. The increases seen at these 3 PPMI clinics are partly driven by increases in staffing, which allowed for increased access to services. In addition, some barriers to access were removed when the constitutional amendment approved by Michigan voters in 2022 was implemented, so the increased demand for abortion seen in these 3 clinics is likely to continue. In addition to the 24-hour waiting period that is currently enjoined, the ban on Medicaid financing for abortion services, as well as the restrictions on commercial insurance coverage for abortion services are being litigated, suggesting financial access to abortion services for Michigan residents might be expanded. Currently, Michigan's Medicaid program provides coverage for prenatal care, childbirth, contraception, and other health services, but not for abortion. The lawsuit argues that, given the 2022 amendment to the

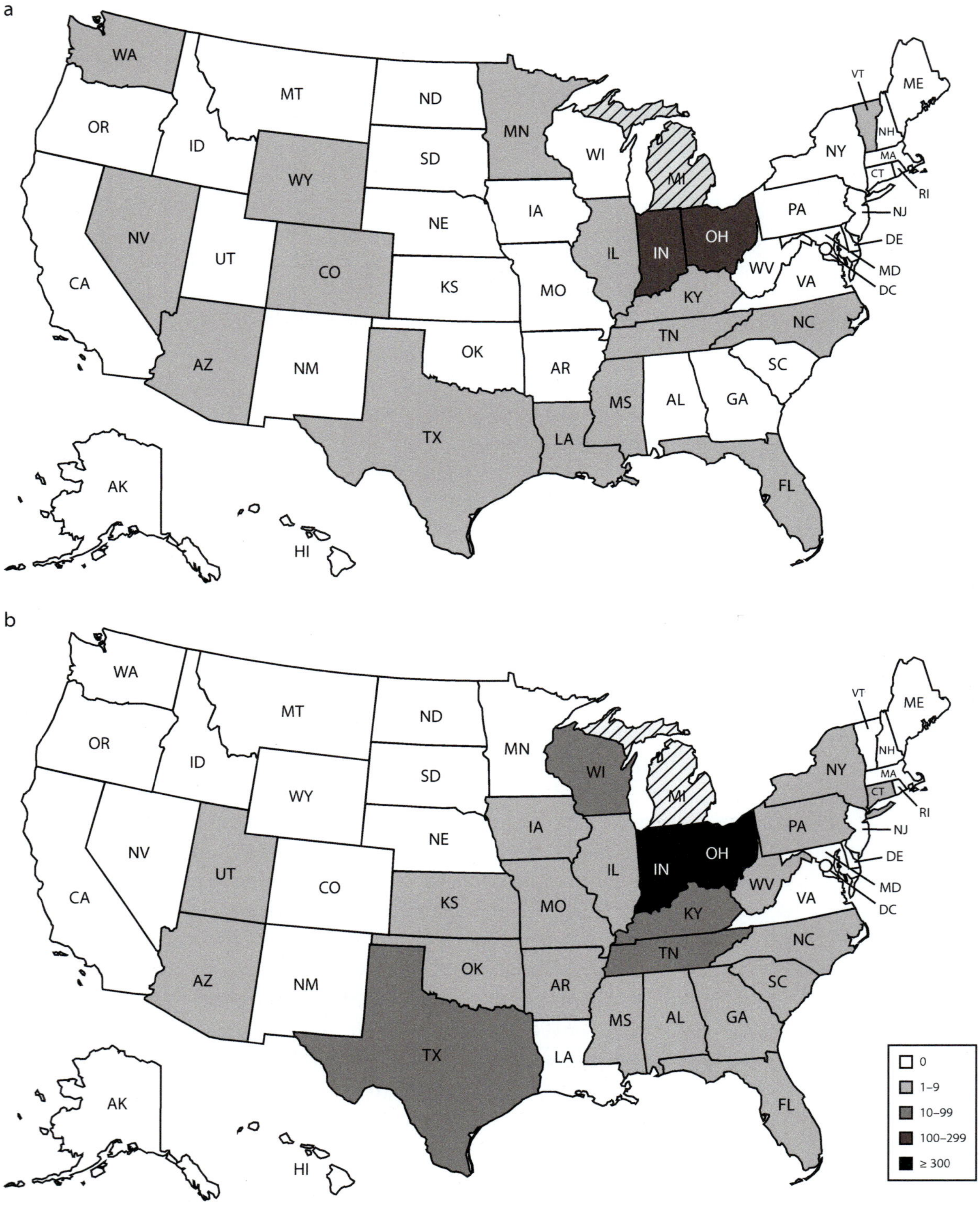

FIGURE 4— **Number of Abortions by State of Residence for Out-of-State Patients Who Received Care at Participating Clinics (a) Before *Dobbs* and (b) After *Dobbs*: United States, July 2021–June 2023**

Note. Maps generated with MapChart. Michigan is marked with diagonal lines as it is the destination state for the study's analysis.

Michigan constitution, the Medicaid program is required to also cover abortion.[23]

The slight decrease in the proportion of medication abortions at these 3 PPMI sites is counter to national trends: by 2020, more than half of abortions nationally were provided via medication,[24] and as of 2023, 63% of abortions in the United States were medication abortions.[25] This reduction in the proportion of medication abortions in our clinics was also seen after *Dobbs* in 2 clinics in Illinois, another surge state that borders states with abortion bans.[14] Conversely, studies from Ohio[9] and Oregon[17] showed that the relative percentage of medication abortion increased after *Dobbs* (in Ohio, it returned to pre-*Dobbs* percentages once the state's 6-week ban was blocked). Simultaneously, we have seen increased accessibility of medication abortion through telehealth services, as evidenced by #WeCount's finding that abortion via telehealth increased from 5% in April to June of 2022 to 25% in October to December of 2024. PPMI similarly has plans to expand their telehealth care, including for abortion.[26] Given that telehealth for abortion is crucial for individuals for whom travel for an in-person abortion would be cumbersome,[27] it is possible that in the future, fewer people may need to travel to a state like Michigan for care.

Limitations

While we believe this analysis has many strengths, there are also important data limitations. Namely, we do not have information about all abortions in Michigan, Michigan residents who may have left the state to access abortion services, changes to the cost of abortion services at these PPMI clinics, or the cost burden felt by clients. In addition, we do not have information about people who were unable to get care or wait times for those who did. There is some speculation that wait times may have increased for Michiganders,[11,21] but our data preclude us from knowing if the increased numbers of patients receiving abortions after 14 weeks gestation were from Michigan or from out of state, and whether these patients sought an abortion earlier in pregnancy but obtained it later because of delays, or whether they were seeking abortion care later in pregnancy. In addition, the aggregate nature of our data means that we cannot explore relationships between the characteristics studied here (e.g., differences in gestation by state of residence) or by other patient characteristics (e.g., age, race). Future studies must rely on chart data or patient surveys to capture this more detailed level of information.

Public Health Implications

At 3 PPMI clinics in southern Michigan, the period following the *Dobbs* decision saw an increase in clinic volume, a rise in the number of patients receiving abortions at later gestational ages, a lower proportion of medication abortions, and an increase in both the proportion of patients coming from out of state and the number of states patients traveled from compared with the same months in the year before *Dobbs*. These observations underscore changes in patient care amid the rapidly evolving abortion landscape in the United States. The post-*Dobbs* landscape, where individuals who need abortion services may have to travel out of state—thereby incurring additional financial and time expenditures—exacerbates existing disparities in access to abortion services, with individuals in restrictive states facing greater barriers to accessing abortion care. To protect the public's health, efforts need to focus on policy advocacy, interstate collaborations, and resource allocation to ensure patients can access the care they need. AJPH

ABOUT THE AUTHORS

Mikaela H. Smith and Alison Norris are with the Division of Epidemiology, School of Public Health, The Ohio State University, Columbus. Caroline Sucher, Vanessa K. Dalton, and Sarah D. Compton are with the Department of Obstetrics and Gynecology, University of Michigan, Ann Arbor.

CORRESPONDENCE

Correspondence should be sent to Sarah D. Compton, 1500 E Medical Center Dr, Ann Arbor, MI 48109 (e-mail: sarahrom@med.umich.edu). Reprints can be ordered at https://www.ajph.org by clicking the "Reprints" link.

PUBLICATION INFORMATION

Full Citation: Smith MH, Sucher C, Norris A, Dalton VK, Compton SD. Examining post-*Dobbs* changes in abortion use at 3 southern Michigan clinics, July 2021–June 2023. *Am J Public Health*. 2026;116(3):351–358.

Acceptance Date: September 25, 2025.

DOI: https://doi.org/10.2105/AJPH.2025.308305

ORCID iDs:

Mikaela H. Smith https://orcid.org/0000-0001-5658-4808

Caroline Sucher https://orcid.org/0009-0000-5048-3264

CONTRIBUTORS

All authors made substantial contributions to the origination or design of the work or the acquisition, analysis, or interpretation of data for the work; drafting the work or revising it critically for important intellectual content; final approval of the version to be published; and agreement to be accountable for all aspects of the work in ensuring that questions related to the accuracy or integrity of any part of the work are appropriately investigated and resolved.

ACKNOWLEDGMENTS

Planned Parenthood Federation of America Inc. reviewed and approved the paper prior to submission.

Note. The findings and conclusions in this article are those of the authors and do not necessarily reflect the views of Planned Parenthood Federation of America Inc.

CONFLICTS OF INTEREST

The authors report no conflicts of interest.

HUMAN PARTICIPANT PROTECTION

This study was approved by the institutional review board at The Ohio State University (IRB 2018H0539). Informed consent was not required because all data used in the study were retrospective and de-identified.

REFERENCES

1. Thompson KMJ, Sturrock HJW, Foster DG, Upadhyay UD. Association of travel distance to nearest abortion facility with rates of abortion. *JAMA Netw Open.* 2021;4(7):e2115530. https://doi.org/10.1001/jamanetworkopen.2021.15530
2. Cartwright AF, Karunaratne M, Barr-Walker J, Johns NE, Upadhyay UD. Identifying national availability of abortion care and distance from major US cities: systematic online search. *J Med Internet Res.* 2018;20(5):e186. https://doi.org/10.2196/jmir.9717
3. Jones RK, Upadhyay UD, Weitz TA. At what cost? Payment for abortion care by US women. *Womens Health Issues.* 2013;23(3):e173–e178. https://doi.org/10.1016/j.whi.2013.03.001
4. Davis MF. The state of abortion rights in the US. *Int J Gynaecol Obstet.* 2022;159(1):324–329. https://doi.org/10.1002/ijgo.14392
5. KFF. Abortion in the United States Dashboard. 2025. Available at: https://www.kff.org/womens-health-policy/dashboard/abortion-in-the-u-s-dashboard. Accessed July 2, 2025.
6. Executive Office of the Governor. Governor Whitmer signs Reproductive Health Act. November 21, 2023. Available at: https://www.michigan.gov/whitmer/news/press-releases/2023/11/21/governor-whitmer-signs-reproductive-health-act. Accessed July 2, 2025.
7. Center for Reproductive Rights. Abortion laws by state. 2025. Available at: https://reproductiverights.org/maps/abortion-laws-by-state. Accessed February 6, 2023.
8. Society of Family Planning. #WeCount report April 2022 to December 2024. 2025. Available at: https://societyfp.org/research/wecount/wecount-december-2024-data. Accessed July 2, 2025.
9. Smith MH, McGowan ML, Kerestes C, Bessett D, Norris AH. Longitudinal impact of *Dobbs v Jackson Women's Health Organization* on abortion service delivery in Ohio, 2022–2023. *Am J Public Health.* 2024;114(10):1034–1042. https://doi.org/10.2105/AJPH.2024.307775
10. Sult A. Indiana Supreme Court rules near-total abortion ban can take effect. ACLU of Indiana. June 30, 2023. Available at: https://www.aclu-in.org/en/press-releases/indiana-supreme-court-rules-near-total-abortion-ban-can-take-effect. Accessed July 2, 2025.
11. Erb R. With Roe overturned, Michigan becomes an abortion 'haven,' for now. *Bridge Michigan.* June 24, 2022. Available at: https://www.bridgemi.com/michigan-health-watch/roe-overturned-michigan-becomes-abortion-haven-now. Accessed October 31, 2024.
12. LeBlanc B. Planned Parenthood expands abortion access in Grand Rapids after repeal of law. *The Detroit News.* March 6, 2024. Available at: https://www.detroitnews.com/story/news/politics/2024/03/06/planned-parenthood-expands-abortion-access-in-grand-rapids/72864950007. Accessed July 2, 2025.
13. The Guttmacher Institute. Monthly Abortion Provision Study. Available at: https://www.guttmacher.org/monthly-abortion-provision-study. Accessed July 2, 2025.
14. Trevino J, Paul R, King E, Reeves JA, Eisenberg DL, Madden T. Abortion trends in Southern Illinois after the *Dobbs v. Jackson Women's Health Organization* decision. *Am J Obstet Gynecol.* 2025; epub ahead of print June 25, 2025. https://doi.org/10.1016/j.ajog.2025.06.046
15. Smith MH, Young D, Dismer H, et al. Clinic adaptations and changes in abortion use after Dobbs in Illinois, July 2021–June 2023. *Am J Public Health.* 2025:e1–e9; epub ahead of print October 16, 2025. https://doi.org/10.2105/AJPH.2025.308273
16. Keefe-Oates B, Fulcher I, Fortin J, et al. Use of abortion services in Massachusetts after the *Dobbs* decision among in-state vs out-of-state residents. *JAMA Netw Open.* 2023;6(9):e2332400. https://doi.org/10.1001/jamanetworkopen.2023.32400
17. Mandelbaum AD, Nacev EC, Fuerst MF, Colwill A, Ramanadhan S, Rodriguez M. Impact of the *Dobbs* decision on abortion services from a large tertiary center in Oregon. *Contraception.* 2024;136:110484. https://doi.org/10.1016/j.contraception.2024.110484
18. Michigan Department of Health and Human Services. Characteristics of induced abortions reported in Michigan. 2023. Available at: https://vitalstats.michigan.gov/osr/abortion/summary.asp. Accessed October 31, 2024.
19. Owda R, Scheerer J, Compton SD, et al. The potential impact of neighboring states' bans on abortion volume in a haven state. *Contraception.* 2023;124:110062. https://doi.org/10.1016/j.contraception.2023.110062
20. White E. Judge blocks Michigan's abortion waiting period, 2 years after voters approved abortion rights. *AP News.* June 25, 2024. Available at: https://apnews.com/article/michigan-abortion-restrictions-injunction-a5b4f582fb621f8730e3209131cb4b90. Accessed October 31, 2024.
21. Erb R. Michigan abortion waits stretch for weeks as out-of-state patients pour in. *Bridge Michigan.* July 29, 2022. Available at: https://www.bridgemi.com/michigan-health-watch/michigan-abortion-waits-stretch-weeks-out-state-patients-pour. Accessed October 31, 2024.
22. Michigan Department of Health and Human Services. Abortion rates for Michigan counties. 2023. Available at: https://vitalstats.michigan.gov/osr/Abortion/AbortionRates.asp. Accessed October 31, 2024.
23. White E. Michigan ban on taxpayer-funded abortions targeted by lawsuit. *AP News.* June 27, 2024. Available at: https://apnews.com/article/michigan-medicaid-abortion-lawsuit-a7489bf8c5c685e78ec5311fe7f1d3a3. Accessed October 31, 2024.
24. Jones RK, Nash E, Cross L, Philbin J, Kirstein M. Medication abortion now accounts for more than half of all US abortions. Guttmacher Institute. February 2022. Available at: https://www.guttmacher.org/article/2022/02/medication-abortion-now-accounts-more-half-all-us-abortions. Accessed October 31, 2024.
25. Jones RK, Friedrich-Karnik A. Medication abortion accounted for 63% of all US abortions in 2023—an increase from 53% in 2020. Guttmacher Institute. March 2024. Available at: https://www.guttmacher.org/2024/03/medication-abortion-accounted-63-all-us-abortions-2023-increase-53-2020. Accessed April 1, 2024.
26. Wells K. Why so many clinics that provide abortion are closing, even where it's still legal. *NPR* May 16, 2025. Available at: https://www.npr.org/sections/shots-health-news/2025/05/16/nx-s1-5397314/planned-parenthood-clinics-abortion-close-telehealth-rights. Accessed July 2, 2025.
27. Donovan MK. Improving access to abortion via telehealth. Guttmacher Institute. May 16, 2019. Available at: https://www.guttmacher.org/gpr/2019/05/improving-access-abortion-telehealth. Accessed October 31, 2024.

Clinic Adaptations and Changes in Abortion Use After *Dobbs* in Illinois, July 2021–June 2023

Mikaela H. Smith, PhD, Danielle Young, MPH, Hanz Dismer, MSW, MPH, Valla Diskin, BS, Lee Hasselbacher, JD, Katherine Rivlin, MD, Danielle Bessett, PhD, and Alison H. Norris, MD, PhD

See also Abortion and Public Health Impact in Post-*Dobbs* Era, pp. 321–367.

Objectives. To assess changes in abortion service delivery in Illinois after the *Dobbs v Jackson Women's Health Organization* decision.

Methods. We used data from a monthly survey of 2 Illinois abortion providers that provide half of Illinois's abortions. We collected data from 2021 to 2023 on abortion counts, overall and stratified by method, gestation duration, and patient state. We compared pre- and post-*Dobbs* findings.

Results. A total of 24 071 abortions took place from July 2021 to June 2022 and 32 579 from July 2022 to June 2023. This 35% increase was driven by a 191% increase in out-of-state patients. Medication abortions increased by 22%, procedural abortions by 53%, and abortions occurring at 12 weeks or later by 75%.

Conclusions. After *Dobbs*, 2 large Illinois abortion providers increasingly offered care to out-of-state patients and patients presenting at later gestations while maintaining in-state abortion rates.

Public Health Implications. Policymakers in states where abortion remains legal can anticipate increased demand for care when other states restrict abortion. By passing legislation to protect access to medication and procedural abortions and abortions later in pregnancy, they can support facilities in meeting patient needs. (*Am J Public Health*. 2026;116(3):359–367. https://doi.org/10.2105/AJPH.2025.308273)

AJPH March 2026, Vol. 116, No. 3

After the 2022 United States Supreme Court decision to overturn *Roe v Wade* in *Dobbs v Jackson Women's Health Organization,* which led to the loss of *Roe*'s federal abortion protections, Illinois has garnered attention as an abortion care safe haven.[1–3] Recent national data from the Society of Family Planning #WeCount project shows Illinois as the state with the largest increase in facility-based abortions in the year after *Dobbs*.[4] Other research from the Guttmacher Institute shows that Illinois saw a 72% increase in clinician-provided abortions in 2023 relative to 2020.[5] However, limited data exist to directly compare monthly changes in characteristics of abortion provision immediately before and after *Dobbs*, including gestation duration, method type, and patient state of residence.

Illinois serves as a useful case study for the role that an abortion-protective state can play in a broader geographic area that is more hostile to abortion. The state has a history of safeguarding abortion access both within and beyond its own borders, including through laws that protect young people's access to care, that expand insurance coverage, and that support patients coming from outside the state (Table A, available as a supplement to the online version of this article at http://www.ajph.org).[1,6–8] In addition to protective policies, the state has dedicated financial resources to patients, including an initiative providing navigation support to patients seeking complex abortion care.[9] Similarly, expansion of Medicaid coverage for abortion in 2018 was associated with decreased disparities in abortion access and more timely care.[10–12]

The relative ease of air and train travel to Chicago, a city with multiple abortion care sites, along with clinics in southern Illinois being proximal to people living in restrictive access states in the Midwest and South (including Arkansas, Indiana, Kentucky, Missouri, and Tennessee), also makes Illinois a likely destination for patients living in these restrictive environments.[13] In addition, Chicago has allocated funds to support abortion seekers and providers and issued an executive order to discourage participation in any investigations.[14]

Along with state policy and state funding, abortion facilities have worked to expand services and infrastructure in the past decade. Several clinics opened facilities or expanded services (including updating facilities so that they could provide procedural abortions and providing additional days of abortion provision) in border cities to offer more access near Missouri, Indiana, Wisconsin, and the southern states.[3,15–18] Notably, the addition of procedural abortion provision to these sites meant that providers could serve patients whose pregnancy was at a later gestational duration than if they provided only medication abortion. Hope Clinic in Granite City, Illinois, just across the state line from St. Louis, Missouri, increased its gestational limit from 23 weeks and 6 days in 2021 to 27 weeks and 5 days in 2023 (personal correspondence, Hope Clinic staff). Planned Parenthood Great Rivers in Missouri also opened a mobile abortion clinic that provided abortion care in Illinois to allow for provision near state borders.[18]

Organizations in Illinois and nearby states have also increased support for patient navigation. Initiatives include abortion funds (e.g., the Chicago Abortion Fund), practical support funds (e.g., funds from the Midwest Access Coalition), a patient navigation program at Planned Parenthood of Illinois (PPIL), and the Regional Logistics Center, a first-of-its-kind partnership between Hope Clinic in Illinois and Planned Parenthood Great Rivers.[19] Investment in community resources such as patient navigation and practical support improves people's ability to access care, and this is true for both those who reside in Illinois and those who travel to Illinois from other states to obtain care.

In this study, we drew on data from an ongoing monthly survey of abortion providers in Illinois to characterize changes in service delivery and abortion use within the state. We describe abortion counts overall and by method, gestational duration, and patient state of residence for the 12 months before and after *Dobbs*. In doing so, we provide insights about changes in abortion care at a critical time point in a key receiving state.

METHODS

We derived the data for this study from an ongoing monthly survey of abortion providers in Illinois. That survey is part of a larger project on abortion provision in several midwestern and southern states.

Data Source

Data collection for our study began in 2020. Our data included monthly overall abortion totals as well as the number of abortions provided via each method (medication or procedural), at each point in gestation (in weeks), and for patients from each state of residence. We included abortions that took place from July 2021 through June 2023 to measure changes in provision in the year preceding and the year following the *Dobbs* decision. These data were provided by 2 large abortion providers in Illinois: Hope Clinic, an independent abortion provider in Granite City in the St. Louis region, and PPIL, which operated 17 health centers throughout central and northern Illinois during the data collection period (Figure 1).

Hope Clinic provides both medication and procedural abortions. At the start of data collection, 5 of the 17 PPIL health centers provided both medication and procedural abortions and 12 provided medication abortions only. Two medication-only sites expanded to include procedural abortions over the course of the study (Figure 1). PPIL began providing medication abortions via telehealth (mailing pills to Illinois addresses) in April 2022, and we included these abortions in our counts of medication abortions.

Each month, a staff member at each participating clinic reported an aggregate of the previous month's abortion volume by method, gestational duration, and patient state of residence. Staff members submitted data through a secure portal using Research Electronic Data Capture (REDCap) tools hosted at Ohio State University.[20,21]

Analysis

Here we present descriptive statistics on monthly abortion volumes. We summed data from all clinics to calculate the numbers and percentages of abortions by method and gestational duration (medication, procedural less than 12 weeks, and procedural 12 weeks or more) and by state of residence (in state vs out of state). We were interested in abortion method given the observed trend of increases in medication abortions over the past decade[22] and the possibility that *Dobbs* might affect access to or availability of medication versus procedural abortions. We defined the pre-*Dobbs* period as July 2021 to June 2022 and the post-*Dobbs* period as July 2022 to June 2023. In addition to ensuring a comparable number of months in each time period, using a full year of data for the pre- and

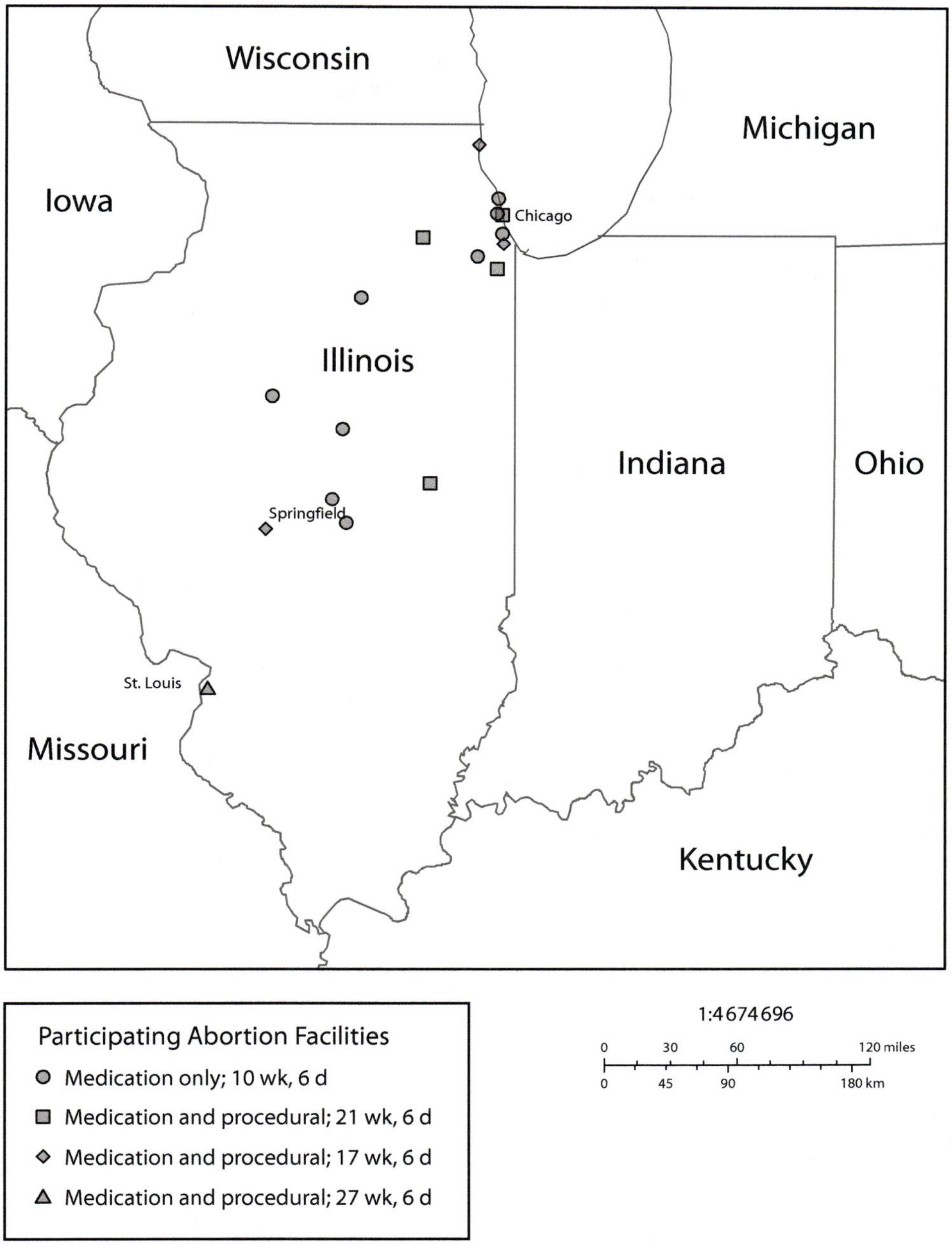

Organization	Methods Provided	Gestation Limit	No. of Sites
Hope Clinic	Medication and procedural	27 wk, 6 d[a]	1
Planned Parenthood of Illinois	Medication and procedural Medication and procedural Medication only	21 wk, 6 d 17 wk, 6 d 10 wk, 6 d	4[b] 3[c] 10–12[d]

FIGURE 1— Abortion Facilities Included in the Study: July 2021–June 2023

[a]Hope incrementally increased its gestational limit, from 23 weeks and 6 days in July 2021 to 24 weeks and 6 days in October 2022, 25 weeks and 6 days in January 2023, and 27 weeks and 6 days in April 2023.
[b]One clinic began providing procedural abortions in September 2022.
[c]One clinic began providing procedural abortions in June 2022.
[d]Because of the addition of procedural abortions in the 2 sites just listed, data represent 12 sites from July 2021 to May 2022, 11 sites from June to August 2022, and 10 sites from September to December 2022.

post-*Dobbs* periods means that the impact of seasonality of abortion care is not the cause of any differences in our comparisons.

We calculated total numbers, monthly means, and percentage changes between the pre-*Dobbs* and post-*Dobbs* periods, comparing method and gestational duration and patient state of residence. Finally, we also calculated, for each state of residence, the number of patients traveling to Illinois in each of the 2 time periods. We analyzed data using Stata version 16 (StataCorp LP, College Station, TX) and created maps using ArcGIS programs (ESRI, Redlands, CA).

RESULTS

The abortions we included represent approximately half of abortions that took place in Illinois during the time period of the study.[23] Overall, from July 2021 to June 2023, the 18 abortion facilities in our study performed 56 650 abortions, or a mean of 2360 abortions per month (Table 1). During the pre-*Dobbs* period (July 2021–June 2022), there were 24 071 abortions, or a mean of 2006 per month. During the post-*Dobbs* period (July 2022–June 2023), there were 32 579 abortions, or a mean of 2715 per month, a 35% increase from before *Dobbs*. Increases in abortion volume began in the 4 months before the *Dobbs* decision, and volume continued to rise after *Dobbs* (Figure 2).

Abortion Method and Gestation Duration

Across the entire study period (July 2021–June 2023), 54% of abortions in Illinois were medication and 46% were procedural (Table 1). The number of medication abortions increased 22% after *Dobbs*, from 13 776 to 16 788, and the number of procedural abortions increased 53%, from 10 305 to 15 791. The 2 facilities that began providing procedural abortions during the study period accounted for about 10% of procedural abortions in the post-*Dobbs* period.

As the total number of procedural abortions rose, procedural abortions occurring before 12 weeks rose by 44% (from 7249 to 10 459), whereas those occurring at 12 weeks or beyond rose by 75% (from 3003 to 5249; Figure A, available as a supplement to the online version of this article at http://www.ajph.org). Abortions occurring at 12 weeks or more as a percentage of all abortions rose from 12% before *Dobbs* (3003 of 24 071) to 16% after *Dobbs* (5249 of 32 579).

State of Residence

Across the study period (July 2021 to June 2023), the number of patients from Illinois stayed consistent while the number of out-of-state patients increased sharply (Figure A). Before *Dobbs*, 81% of patients (19 666) were from Illinois and 19% (4477) were from outside of the state. After *Dobbs*, 60% of patients were from Illinois (19 633) and 40% (13 044) were from outside Illinois, reflecting a 191% increase in out-of-state patients. Both before and after *Dobbs* (Table 2), the highest percentages of patients came to Illinois from Missouri (57% before, 27% after), Indiana (15% before, 10% after), and Wisconsin (8% before, 22% after). The greatest increases from before *Dobbs* to after *Dobbs* in patients traveling to Illinois were among those from Wisconsin (from 351 to 2840 patients), Tennessee (from 140 to 1775 patients), Missouri (from 2571 to 3519 patients), Indiana (from 664 to 1316 patients), and Arkansas (from 88 to 605 patients).

DISCUSSION

After the *Dobbs* decision, abortion care provided by 2 large abortion providers in Illinois was marked by increased numbers of abortions, increased use of procedural abortions, and greater proportions of patients having abortions at 12 weeks or beyond. Illinois, already a state to which patients traveled before *Dobbs*, became even more of a haven state for out-of-state patients after *Dobbs*. We found that the number of abortions provided at participating facilities increased by 35%, with the increase resulting from the almost tripling volume of out-of-state patients.

Our finding of this 35% increase in abortions after *Dobbs* is slightly lower than the 40% increase in Illinois's monthly number of abortions reported by #WeCount. Specifically, #WeCount documented 5570 abortions per month before *Dobbs* (average of April and May 2022) and 7807 abortions per month after *Dobbs* (average of April, May, and June 2023).[24] This comparison suggests that other clinics in the state also saw large increases in patient load. Similarly, the Guttmacher Institute's Monthly Abortion Provision Study reported an increase in abortions in Illinois from 52 780 in 2020 to 90 900 in 2023.[5] This represents a 72% increase in patient numbers, much larger than our 35% increase; however, because the Guttmacher study's comparison year was 2020, the 72% increase also represents increases in patient numbers in the years leading up to *Dobbs*.[25]

The decrease in number of abortions between September and December 2022, as compared with earlier in 2022, is paralleled in national data[24] and may be reflective of normal seasonal trends in abortion demand and provision.

TABLE 1— Numbers of Abortions at 18 Abortion Facilities in Illinois and Breakdown by Method, Gestation, In-State Versus Out-of-State Patient Residence, and Month: Illinois, July 2021 to June 2023

	Total, No. (%)	Medication, No. (%)	Procedural, No. (%)	Procedural <12 Weeks, No. (%)	Procedural ≥12 Weeks, No. (%)	In State, No. (%)	Out of State, No. (%)
Before *Dobbs*							
July 2021	1931 (100)	968 (50)	963 (50)	730 (38)	220 (11)	1601 (83)	335 (17)
August 2021	1807 (100)	1028 (57)	779 (43)	562 (31)	211 (12)	1549 (85)	265 (15)
September 2021	1937 (100)	1049 (54)	888 (46)	634 (33)	249 (13)	1623 (84)	314 (16)
October 2021	1772 (100)	930 (52)	842 (48)	611 (34)	216 (12)	1475 (83)	296 (17)
November 2021	1585 (100)	928 (59)	657 (41)	482 (30)	169 (11)	1303 (82)	277 (18)
December 2021	1771 (100)	1063 (60)	708 (40)	491 (28)	210 (12)	1451 (82)	326 (18)
January 2022	2033 (100)	1190 (59)	843 (41)	575 (28)	268 (13)	1653 (80)	407 (20)
February 2022	1926 (100)	1103 (57)	823 (43)	543 (28)	280 (15)	1596 (82)	350 (18)
March 2022	2349 (100)	1376 (59)	973 (41)	652 (28)	321 (14)	1888 (80)	478 (20)
April 2022	2225 (100)	1363 (61)	862 (39)	578 (26)	284 (13)	1823 (81)	421 (19)
May 2022	2243 (100)	1361 (61)	882 (39)	605 (27)	277 (12)	1827 (81)	430 (19)
June 2022	2492 (100)	1407 (56)	1085 (44)	786 (32)	298 (12)	1877 (76)	578 (24)
Total	24071 (100)	13766 (57)	10305 (43)	7249 (30)	3003 (12)	19666 (81)	4477 (19)
Mean	2006	1147	859	604	250	1639	373
After *Dobbs*							
July 2022	2740 (100)	1385 (51)	1355 (49)	888 (32)	467 (17)	1542 (56)	1227 (44)
August 2022	3060 (100)	1708 (56)	1352 (44)	899 (29)	452 (15)	1870 (61)	1205 (39)
September 2022	2571 (100)	1348 (52)	1223 (48)	819 (32)	382 (15)	1482 (58)	1094 (42)
October 2022	2688 (100)	1368 (51)	1320 (49)	887 (33)	426 (16)	1604 (59)	1094 (41)
November 2022	2006 (100)	1001 (50)	1005 (50)	627 (31)	363 (18)	1130 (57)	870 (44)
December 2022	2619 (100)	1339 (51)	1280 (49)	839 (32)	427 (16)	1593 (61)	1027 (39)
January 2023	2829 (100)	1382 (49)	1447 (51)	910 (32)	537 (19)	1752 (62)	1077 (38)
February 2023	2736 (100)	1393 (51)	1343 (49)	872 (32)	476 (17)	1701 (62)	1044 (38)
March 2023	3066 (100)	1642 (54)	1424 (46)	941 (31)	483 (16)	1884 (61)	1190 (39)
April 2023	2727 (100)	1371 (50)	1356 (50)	916 (34)	413 (15)	1680 (61)	1057 (39)
May 2023	2771 (100)	1492 (54)	1279 (46)	876 (32)	403 (15)	1688 (61)	1088 (39)
June 2023	2766 (100)	1359 (49)	1407 (51)	985 (36)	420 (15)	1707 (61)	1071 (39)
Total	32579 (100)	16788 (52)	15791 (48)	10459 (32)	5249 (16)	19633 (60)	13044 (40)
Mean	2715	1399	1316	872	437	1636	1087
Overall total, %	56650 (100)	30554 (54)	26096 (46)	17708 (31)	8252 (15)	39299 (69)	17521 (31)
Mean	2360	1273	1087	738	344	1637	730

Note. Dobbs = *Dobbs v Jackson Women's Health Organization*. Sums by gestation may not equal total procedural abortions and sums by state of residence may not equal total reported abortions.

The drop in volume in November was likely also driven by a complex and resource-intensive transition of electronic medical record systems at PPIL. Capacity has been shown to decrease during similar transitions in other specialties.[26,27] Although abortion providers are susceptible to the same operational challenges as other health care providers (e.g., changes in infrastructure, staff turnover), they have experienced these challenges amid a uniquely demanding and changing abortion policy landscape.

It is noteworthy that the use of medication abortions increased in absolute numbers but decreased as a percentage of all abortions after *Dobbs* (from 57% to 52%). The absolute increase in the number of medication abortions and the relatively greater increase in

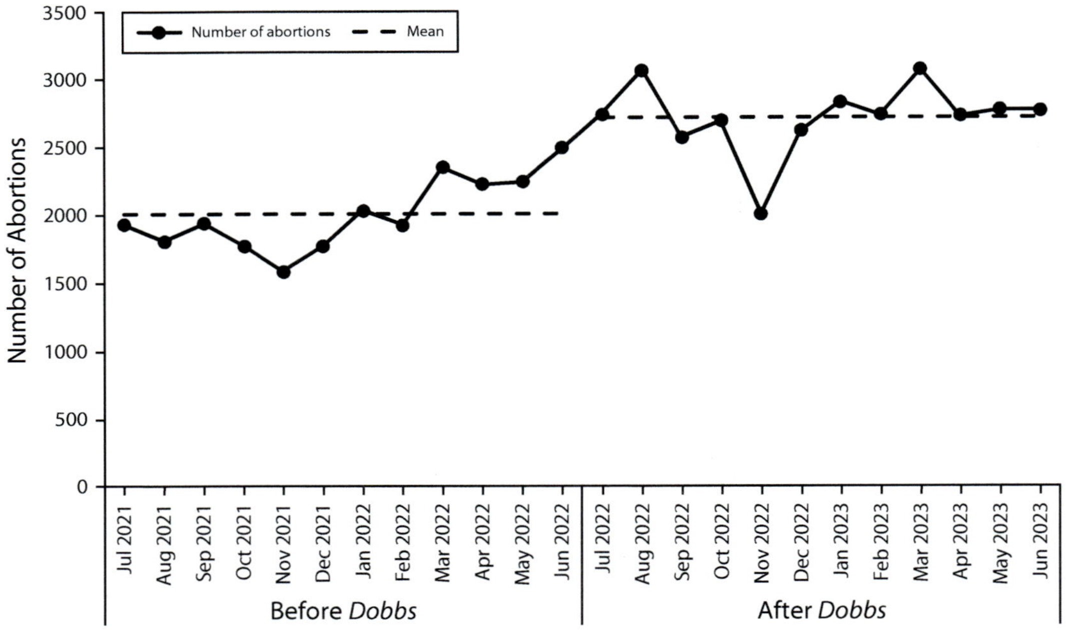

FIGURE 2— Numbers of Abortions at 18 Abortion Facilities in Illinois: July 2021–June 2023

Note. Dobbs = Dobbs v Jackson Women's Health Organization.

AJPH March 2026, Vol. 116, No. 3

the number and proportion of procedural abortions could be related to several factors, including patient preference, expansion of procedural services at 2 PPIL clinics, and increased gestation duration owing to travel-related delays. However, our data preclude a further understanding of what motivated this change. Previous research shows that some patients prefer medication abortions and some prefer procedural abortions[28] and that there are nuances in these preferences,[29] highlighting the importance of expansion of access to both types of abortions in states working to protect access. Given that increasing proportions of patients across the United States are using medication abortions, it is notable that among the clinics in our sample the proportion of medication abortions decreased over the study period.

It is also worth mentioning that the percentage of abortions at 12 weeks or later increased after *Dobbs*, from 12% to 16%. Given that the large majority of abortions in the United States occur earlier in pregnancy (93% of all abortions in 2022 occurred at or before 13 weeks of gestation),[25] this increase in Illinois is meaningful. This finding has important implications given that abortion later in gestation can be more expensive and can involve higher medical risks for patients, so patient care may be more complex for patients presenting later in gestation.[30] This increase could be related to expansion of services (such as Hope increasing its gestational limit or PPIL adding procedural abortion provision at 2 of its sites) or to the consequences of overcoming barriers experienced by people traveling from out of state for abortion care, but our data cannot provide an explanation of why or for which groups the increase occurred.

We observed almost a 3-fold increase in travel to Illinois among out-of-state patients, whereas provision of in-state abortions remained relatively consistent. Our findings align with those of the Guttmacher Institute, which estimated that the percentage of patients coming from out of the state into Illinois increased from 21% in 2020 to 41% in 2023.[5] On the eve of the *Dobbs* decision, many stakeholders were concerned that influxes of out-of-state patients would overwhelm the receiving state abortion care systems. Our data show that in Illinois, where there was a significant increase in out-of-state patients, clinics maintained a consistent volume of care for state residents. Finally, out-of-state travel, although demonstrating success in terms of patients being able to obtain needed abortion care, is burdensome and disproportionately difficult for people with structural disadvantages.[31]

The highest percentages of patients traveling to Illinois both before and after *Dobbs* were from Missouri, Indiana, and Wisconsin, all of which share a

TABLE 2— Numbers of Abortion Patients by Patient State of Residence Before Versus After *Dobbs*: Illinois, July 2021–June 2023

State	Before *Dobbs*	After *Dobbs*	Change, No. (%)
Alabama	3	111	108 (3600)
Alaska	0	1	1 (. . .)
Arizona	2	124	122 (6100)
Arkansas	88	605	517 (588)
California	4	3	−1 (−25)
Colorado	1	2	1 (100)
Connecticut	3	0	−3 (. . .)
Florida	4	70	66 (1650)
Georgia	4	68	64 (1600)
Hawaii	0	1	1 (. . .)
Indiana	664	1316	652 (98)
Iowa	66	159	93 (141)
Kansas	17	51	34 (200)
Kentucky	117	543	426 (364)
Louisiana	13	242	229 (1762)
Maryland	1	0	−1 (. . .)
Massachusetts	0	3	3 (. . .)
Michigan	31	45	14 (45)
Minnesota	6	6	0 (0)
Mississippi	34	522	488 (1435)
Missouri	2571	3519	948 (37)
Montana	2	0	−2 (. . .)
Nebraska	2	3	1 (50)
Nevada	1	2	1 (100)
New Hampshire	1	0	−1 (. . .)
New Jersey	0	2	2 (. . .)
New York	3	3	0 (0)
North Carolina	1	0	−1 (. . .)
Ohio	36	291	255 (708)
Oklahoma	19	78	59 (311)
Oregon	1	0	−1 (. . .)
Pennsylvania	2	3	1 (50)
South Carolina	2	4	2 (100)
South Dakota	1	1	0 (0)
Tennessee	140	1775	1635 (1168)
Texas	162	608	446 (275)
Vermont	0	1	1 (. . .)
Virginia	4	3	−1 (−25)
Washington	1	0	−1 (. . .)
Wisconsin	351	2840	2489 (709)

Note. Dobbs = *Dobbs v Jackson Women's Health Organization*. No patients from Delaware, Idaho, Maine, New Mexico, North Dakota, Rhode Island, Utah, West Virginia, Wyoming, or the District of Columbia traveled to Illinois in either time period.

border with Illinois. After *Dobbs,* abortion was banned in Missouri and Wisconsin (and eventually Indiana, although after our study time period),[7] and there were increases in the numbers of patients from Missouri (by 37%), Indiana (by 98%), and Wisconsin (by 709%). Abortion was also banned in states farther from Illinois, such as Arkansas, Kentucky, Mississippi, Tennessee, and Texas,[7] and more than 400 additional patients came from each of those states after *Dobbs*. Our findings thus highlight the role that Illinois played as a haven state for patients who traveled huge distances.

Limitations and Strengths

Overall, our ability to compare pre- and post-*Dobbs* data among the same facilities and over the same months strengthens our ability to interpret the impact of the *Dobbs* decision. Our study is limited because we do not have data from all abortion providers in Illinois, and thus changes in service delivery or the number of abortions occurring at other clinics are not reflected in our findings. Illinois does not report data on method and gestational duration to the US Centers for Disease Control and Prevention Abortion Surveillance System,[25] so we cannot know how our findings compare with statewide trends.

In addition, given that our data drew from abortion providers with locations in the southern part of the state, our findings may reflect a higher proportion of out-of-state travelers relative to other clinics in Illinois. Illinois is uniquely situated both geographically and politically, so it is also possible that the policies and practices that have been important in supporting access to care in Illinois may not translate to other states. Moreover, our data cannot speak to those

AJPH March 2026, Vol. 116, No. 3

who attempted, and failed, to obtain care in Illinois. Because our data are aggregate counts, we cannot further refine differences in, for example, method and gestational duration by state of residence, which would shed important light on whether the burdens associated with traveling from out of the state led to patients receiving abortions at later gestational points.

Finally, without additional demographic information about patients, we are not able to assess the potential inequities in abortion access that might be reflected in our findings. People with lower incomes and less education and people of color experience additional burdens related to receiving abortion care,[32–34] but our data cannot speak to such differences.

Public Health Implications

When people in states that restrict abortion are left without or with limited access to services, many travel out of state to obtain care.[5] The increase in people traveling from out of state shows Illinois's critical role in making abortion access a reality for people across the United States, particularly midwesterners and southerners. Policymakers in states in which abortion remains legal can support access to abortion care for both in-state and out-of-state residents by passing legislation to facilitate patient needs. These needs include affordability: states that allow Medicaid funds to be used for abortion free up resources from local abortion funds to support a larger number of patients, including those coming from out of state.[12] Laws that support expanded access to medication and procedural abortions as well as abortions later in pregnancy will lead to improved patient health and well-being.[35] AJPH

ABOUT THE AUTHORS

Mikaela H. Smith and Alison H. Norris are with the Division of Epidemiology, College of Public Health, The Ohio State University, Columbus. At the time of the study, Danielle Young was with Planned Parenthood of Illinois, Chicago. Hanz Dismer and Valla Diskin are with Hope Clinic, Granite City, IL. Lee Hasselbacher and Katherine Rivlin are with the Department of Obstetrics & Gynecology, University of Chicago Medicine, Chicago, IL. Danielle Bessett is with the Sociology Department, University of Cincinnati, Cincinnati, OH.

CORRESPONDENCE

Correspondence should be sent to Mikaela H. Smith, PhD, 250 Cunz Hall, 1841 Neil Ave, Columbus, OH 43210 (e-mail: smith.14017@osu.edu). Reprints can be ordered at http://www.ajph.org by clicking the "Reprints" link.

PUBLICATION INFORMATION

Full Citation: Smith MH, Young D, Dismer H, et al. Clinic adaptations and changes in abortion use after *Dobbs* in Illinois, July 2021–June 2023. *Am J Public Health*. 2026;116(3):359–367.

Acceptance Date: August 12, 2025.

DOI: https://doi.org/10.2105/AJPH.2025.308273

ORCID iDs:

Mikaela H. Smith https://orcid.org/0000-0001-5658-4808

Danielle Young https://orcid.org/0009-0005-8051-5892

Hanz Dismer https://orcid.org/0009-0000-5089-6288

CONTRIBUTORS

M. H. Smith contributed to conceptualization, data curation, analysis, project administration, visualization, writing, and reviewing. D. Young, H. Dismer, and V. Diskin contributed to data curation, analysis, validation, writing, and reviewing. L. Hasselbacher and K. Rivlin contributed to analysis, writing, and reviewing. D. Bessett contributed to analysis, supervision, writing, and reviewing. A. H. Norris contributed to conceptualization, analysis, supervision, writing, and reviewing.

ACKNOWLEDGMENTS

This study was funded by a grant from a philanthropic foundation that makes grants anonymously. Support for this project was also provided by the Ohio State University Institute for Population Research through grant P2CHD058484 from the Eunice Kennedy Shriver National Institute of Child Health and Human Development of the National Institutes of Health. The Research Electronic Data Capture tool used for data collection was supported by the National Center for Advancing Translational Sciences (grant UL1TR001070).

Note. The content is solely the responsibility of the authors and does not necessarily represent the official views of the Eunice Kennedy Shriver National Institute of Child Health and Human Development, the National Institutes of Health, or the Planned Parenthood Federation of America Inc.

CONFLICTS OF INTEREST

The authors have no conflicts of interest to disclose.

HUMAN PARTICIPANT PROTECTION

This study was approved by the institutional review boards of The Ohio State University and the University of Cincinnati.

REFERENCES

1. Illinois.gov. Gov. Pritzker signs sweeping reproductive rights protections into law. Available at: https://www.illinois.gov/news/press-release.25906.html. Accessed March 17, 2024.
2. Lang M. One year after Roe v. Wade's overturn: Illinois emerges as abortion care safe haven. Available at: https://newschannel20.com/news/local/one-year-after-roe-v-wades-overturn-illinois-emerges-as-abortion-care-safe-haven. Accessed March 17, 2024.
3. Kenning C. How one quiet Illinois college town became the symbol of abortion rights in America. Available at: https://www.usatoday.com/in-depth/news/investigations/2023/06/04/carbondale-illinois-abortion-clinics/70180040007. Accessed August 16, 2023.
4. Society of Family Planning. #WeCount report April 2022 to December 2023. Available at: https://societyfp.org/wp-content/uploads/2024/05/WeCount-report-6-May-2024-Dec-2023-data_Final.pdf. Accessed August 16, 2023.
5. Maddow-Zimet I, Philbin J, DoCampo I, Jones RK. Monthly Abortion Provision Study. Available at: https://osf.io/k4x7t. Accessed December 7, 2023.
6. Lourgos AL, Rumore K. Timeline: abortion funding in Illinois from Medicaid to the Reproductive Health Act. Available at: https://www.chicagotribune.com/2022/06/24/timeline-abortion-funding-in-illinois-from-medicaid-to-the-reproductive-health-act. Accessed March 17, 2024.
7. Guttmacher Institute. Interactive map: US abortion policies and access after Roe. Available at: https://states.guttmacher.org/policies. Accessed June 14, 2023.
8. Center for Reproductive Rights. Abortion laws by state: Illinois. Available at: https://reproductiverights.org/maps/state/illinois. Accessed July 8, 2024.
9. Schorsch K. Illinois governor JB Pritzker is launching a hotline to help high-risk patients get abortions at hospitals. Available at: https://www.wbez.org/stories/illinois-launching-hotline-for-high-risk-abortion-help/e6674b6d-0c15-452e-9f25-7bffb5472f92. July 31, 2023. Accessed August 16, 2023.
10. Zuniga C, Bommaraju A, Hasselbacher L, Stulberg D, Thompson TA. Provider and community stakeholder perspectives of expanding Medicaid coverage of abortion in Illinois. *BMC Health Serv Res*. 2022;22(1):413. https://doi.org/10.1186/s12913-022-07761-5
11. Zuniga C, Hernandez V, Stulberg D, et al. Changes in abortion access after implementation of Medicaid coverage in Illinois: a retrospective analysis.

BMJ Public Health. 2025;3(1):e001966. https://doi.org/10.1136/bmjph-2024-001966

12. Heil SKR, Caglayan K, Castillo G, et al. The impact of state Medicaid coverage of abortion on people accessing care in three states. *Perspect Sex Reprod Health*. 2024;56(3):255–268. https://doi.org/10.1111/psrh.12275
13. Samee Ali S. Illinois abortion clinics see ripple effects of Roe reversal as surrounding states implement bans. Available at: https://www.nbcnews.com/news/us-news/illinois-abortion-clinics-see-ripple-effects-roe-reversal-surrounding-rcna35946?cid=sm_npd_nn_tw_ma. Accessed March 17, 2024.
14. Chicago Department of Public Health. Abortion care. Available at: https://www.chicago.gov/content/city/en/depts/cdph/provdrs/healthy_families/svcs/abortion-care.html. Accessed June 9, 2025.
15. Corley C. Illinois is preparing for a potential influx of people seeking abortions. Available at: https://www.npr.org/2022/05/09/1097540931/illinois-influx-seeking-abortions-roe-v-wade. Accessed August 16, 2023.
16. Schorsch K. Abortion is legal in Illinois. In Wisconsin, it's nearly banned. So clinics teamed up. Available at: https://www.npr.org/sections/health-shots/2022/08/11/1114647820/illinois-wisconsin-abortions. Accessed August 16, 2023.
17. Simmons E. Champaign Planned Parenthood adds in-clinic abortions after Indiana's ban. Available at: https://www.news-gazette.com/news/local/health-care/champaign-planned-parenthood-adds-in-clinic-abortions-after-indianas-ban/article_009de6e2-7ee7-5a6b-8dd8-7561bde9bf2d.html. Accessed March 17, 2024.
18. McCammon S. Planned Parenthood mobile clinic will take abortion to red-state borders. Available at: https://www.npr.org/2022/10/03/1125797779/planned-parenthood-mobile-clinic-will-take-abortion-to-red-state-borders. Accessed August 16, 2023.
19. Early R. CBS and Harper's Bazaar praise St. Louis area abortion access center. Available at: https://www.riverfronttimes.com/news/cbs-and-harpers-bazaar-praise-st-louis-area-abortion-access-center-37673859. Accessed March 17, 2024.
20. Harris PA, Taylor R, Thielke R, Payne J, Gonzalez N, Conde JG. Research Electronic Data Capture (REDCap)—a metadata-driven methodology and workflow process for providing translational research informatics support. *J Biomed Inform*. 2009;42(2):377–381. https://doi.org/10.1016/cksdbv
21. Harris PA, Taylor R, Minor BL, et al. The REDCap Consortium: building an international community of software platform partners. *J Biomed Inform*. 2019;95:103208. https://doi.org/10.1016/ggqm7d
22. Jones RK, Friedrich-Karnik A. Medication abortion accounted for 63% of all US abortions in 2023—an increase from 53% in 2020. Available at: https://www.guttmacher.org/2024/03/medication-abortion-accounted-63-all-us-abortions-2023-increase-53-2020. Accessed April 1, 2024.
23. Illinois Department of Public Health. Abortion statistics. Available at: https://dph.illinois.gov/data-statistics/vital-statistics/abortion-statistics.html. Accessed January 23, 2024.
24. Society of Family Planning. #WeCount report April 2022 through June 2024. Available at: https://societyfp.org/wp-content/uploads/2024/10/WeCount-Report-8-June-2024-data.pdf. Accessed January 23, 2024.
25. Centers for Disease Control and Prevention. CDC's Abortion Surveillance System FAQs. Available at: https://www.cdc.gov/reproductive-health/data-statistics/abortion-surveillance-system.html. Accessed August 1, 2024.
26. Huang C, Koppel R, McGreevey JD, Craven CK, Schreiber R. Transitions from one electronic health record to another: challenges, pitfalls, and recommendations. *Appl Clin Inform*. 2020;11(5):742–754. https://doi.org/10.1055/s-0040-1718535
27. Haidar YM, Moshtaghi O, Mahboubi H, et al. Association between electronic medical record implementation and otolaryngologist productivity in the ambulatory setting. *JAMA Otolaryngol Head Neck Surg*. 2017;143(1):20–24. https://doi.org/10.1001/jamaoto.2016.2528
28. Turner T, Quasebarth M, Boesche M, Moore A, Stulberg DB, Hasselbacher LA. "I knew which one I wanted": interviews with Illinois patients to explore abortion method decision-making after insurance expansion. *Reprod Female Child Health*. 2024;56(2):99–107. https://doi.org/10.1002/rfc2.66
29. Thomas K, Bornstein M, Odum T, Bessett D, Turner AN, Rivlin K. Who gets the abortion method they prefer? *Contraception*. 2024;134:110412. https://doi.org/10.1016/j.contraception.2024.110412
30. Raymond EG, Grimes DA. The comparative safety of legal induced abortion and childbirth in the United States. *Obstet Gynecol*. 2012;119(2):215–219. https://doi.org/10.1097/AOG.0b013e31823fe923
31. Chakraborty P, Murawsky S, Smith MH, McGowan ML, Norris AH, Bessett D. How Ohio's proposed abortion bans would impact travel distance to access abortion care. *Perspect Sex Reprod Health*. 2022;54(2):54–63. https://doi.org/10.1363/psrh.12191
32. Dehlendorf C, Harris LH, Weitz TA. Disparities in abortion rates: a public health approach. *Am J Public Health*. 2013;103(10):1772–1779. https://doi.org/10.2105/AJPH.2013.301339
33. Turner AN, Brenner-Levoy J, Rivlin K, et al. Who loses access to legal abortion with a 6-week ban? *Am J Obstet Gynecol*. 2022;227(5):777–780. https://doi.org/10.1016/j.ajog.2022.06.032
34. Redd SK, Mosley EA, Narasimhan S, et al. Estimation of multiyear consequences for abortion access in Georgia under a law limiting abortion to early pregnancy. *JAMA Netw Open*. 2023;6(3):e231598. https://doi.org/10.1001/jamanetworkopen.2023.1598
35. Foster DG. *The Turnaway Study: Ten Years, a Thousand Women, and the Consequences of Having—or Being Denied—an Abortion*. Scribner; 2020.

Validating Georgia's Vaccine Registry for the COVID-19 2023–2024 Season: True GRITS

Allison D. Roebling, DVM, MPH, Nathaniel Elijah Barrera-Nitz, MPH, Melissa Tobin-D'Angelo, MD, MPH, Kyle P. Openo, DrPH, and Lucy S. Witt, MD, MPH, MSc

Objectives. To determine the completeness of providers' COVID-19 vaccine reporting to the Georgia Registry of Immunization Transactions and Services between October 1, 2023, and December 31, 2023.

Methods. We performed active, population, and laboratory surveillance in metropolitan Atlanta, Georgia, to identify all residents hospitalized with COVID-19. We selected a subset of patients by using age-stratified random sampling. We telephoned patients or their proxies, pharmacies, and primary care physicians to verify vaccination status and obtain date of unrecorded vaccination (if applicable) for cases without recorded vaccination on or after September 1, 2023.

Results. In the 8-county metro Atlanta catchment area, 2165 patients were hospitalized for COVID-19 during the study period, with 135 patients sampled for full chart reviews. Eighty-six patients required follow-up calls, resulting in 525 telephone calls and approximately 120 person-hours. From follow-up, we identified only 1 vaccine dose not in the registry.

Conclusions. The registry is relatively reliable for obtaining information on COVID-19 vaccination status for patients in metropolitan Atlanta. Additional follow-up does not elucidate additional information. (*Am J Public Health*. 2026;116(3):368–371. https://doi.org/10.2105/AJPH.2025.308325)

AJPH March 2026, Vol. 116, No. 3

The Emerging Infections Program (EIP) is a network of 12 US sites that perform active population-based infectious disease surveillance coordinated and funded via the Centers for Disease Control and Prevention.[1] The Georgia EIP is a collaboration between the Georgia Department of Public Health, Emory University, and the Atlanta Veterans Administration Medical Center. For EIP's COVID-19 Hospitalization Surveillance Network (COVID-NET) program, trained surveillance officers collect data in a standardized case report form on patients hospitalized with severe acute respiratory syndrome coronavirus 2 infections.[2] Study sites use state immunization information systems (IISs) to determine patient vaccination status, with additional follow-up if the state IIS is unreliable. To determine whether Georgia's IIS was reliable for COVID-19 vaccination status, we initiated a study by using vaccine follow-up calls to find missing doses.

METHODS

In Georgia, COVID-NET patients are defined as residents of an 8-county metro Atlanta catchment area who are admitted as inpatients to a hospital and test positive for COVID-19 either during their hospital stay or in the 14 days before hospitalization. Our study included an age-stratified sample of patients, as determined by Centers for Disease Control and Prevention COVID-NET guidance, with an admission date from October 1, 2023, to December 31, 2023. Sampled patients received vaccine follow-up calls unless (1) they had documentation of a vaccination in the Georgia Registry of Immunization and Transaction Services (GRITS, the state IIS)[3] on or after September 1, 2023 (n = 8), (2) their medical record explicitly stated that they were unvaccinated for COVID-19 (n = 23), or (3) they were ineligible for vaccination because they were younger than 6 months (n = 18).

We telephoned primary care providers (PCPs), pharmacies, and patients or patient proxies (i.e., parents, spouses, or other emergency contacts) contingent on the availability of contact information. Follow-up consisted of 3 call attempts to PCPs, 3 call attempts to pharmacies, and 5 call attempts to patients or proxies. We collected data on vaccine doses received between September 1, 2022, and hospitalization.

Vaccine follow-up efforts fell into the following categories:

1. The source could not be reached, refused to provide information, or was unable to provide information on vaccination status.
2. The source was not aware of any vaccination, or there was no record of patient vaccination.
3. The source verified that the patient was unvaccinated.
4. The source provided information on a vaccine dose already in GRITS.
5. The source reported that vaccines were given but were not in GRITS.

We calculated descriptive statistics for each category and stratified them by whether the patient had a vaccine dose recorded in GRITS between September 1, 2022, and August 31, 2023.

RESULTS

The Georgia COVID-NET recorded 2165 patients from the catchment area who were hospitalized with COVID-19 with admission dates from October 1 through December 31, 2023. Of these, we sampled 135 for full chart reviews. Additional follow-up was required for 86 (63.7%) patients to confirm COVID-19 vaccine status and obtain any potentially missed vaccinations.

Follow-Up

There was no contact information for PCPs in their medical records for 25 of 86 (29%) patients. Of the PCPs we contacted, 29 (48%) could not provide additional information. Three PCPs confirmed that the patients were unvaccinated, but 1 reported a vaccine dose administered by a pharmacy that was not in GRITS (Table 1).

Follow-up with pharmacies yielded the least additional information. There was no pharmacy information in their medical records for 17 (20%) patients, and the remaining contacted pharmacies provided no new or additional information.

Most often, follow-up with patients or proxies yielded no information, either because no one answered the calls or the person answering was unwilling or unable to provide additional vaccine information (71 of 86 cases; Table 1). Fourteen (18%) patients or their proxies verified that the patients were unvaccinated at the time of their hospitalization. No patients or proxies provided a previously unreported vaccine dose.

Final Status

After we made additional contacts with sources, we identified only 1 previously unknown vaccine. Most follow-up calls provided no additional information. We verified 17 (22%) patients as unvaccinated who were presumed unvaccinated before follow-up calls (Table 1). We were unable to contact any sources by any method for 9 patients. In total, we made 525 call attempts to verify COVID-19 vaccination status for 86 patients; this took approximately 120 person-hours and yielded only 1 previously undocumented vaccine dose.

DISCUSSION

IISs are computerized databases in which all participating providers can enter and view vaccine doses for residents of a specific geographic area.[4,5] All 50 US states receive federal funding to maintain an IIS for public health surveillance and patient care continuity, but data completeness in these databases varies.[4] A 2008 study in Arizona found 59% agreement between PCP charts and IISs on vaccine information for pediatric patients,[6] whereas a 2006 study in Philadelphia, Pennsylvania, found that vaccine coverage for pediatric patients was 18% lower in the state IIS versus PCP charts.[7] In Georgia, providers are required by law to enter vaccines into GRITS, but compliance has been inconsistent and patients may opt out of participation.[8,9]

Early in the COVID-19 pandemic, federal regulations for vaccine access required that any providers administering COVID-19 vaccines report these vaccines to IISs.[10,11] This increased reliability of IIS data for COVID-19 vaccine receipt: a 2023 study found 94.5% of providers in compliance with IIS reporting requirements.[11] Federal oversight of IIS reporting expired for COVID-19 vaccines in October 2023.[10] Following this change, the Georgia EIP initiated vaccine follow-up calls to determine whether GRITS had become less reliable for evaluating COVID-19 vaccination status in our study population.

Follow-up calls to verify patients' vaccination status and obtain missing vaccination data for 86 patients hospitalized with COVID-19 between September 1, 2023, and December 30, 2023, did not yield significant additional information. We found Georgia's state IIS (GRITS) to be relatively reliable for

TABLE 1— Results of Follow-Up Calls to Determine COVID-19 Vaccination Status by Information Source and Vaccination Status Between September 1, 2022, and August 31, 2023, in GRITS

	Patients With COVID-19 Vaccination in GRITS (n = 7), No. (%)	Patients Without COVID-19 Vaccination in GRITS (n = 79), No. (%)	Total (n = 86), No. (%)
Primary care physicians contact attempts	3	58	61
No information could be provided	2 (67)	27 (47)	29 (48)
No record of vaccinations	0	28 (48)	28 (46)
Verified unvaccinated	0	3 (5)	3 (5)
Verified vaccines already in GRITS	0	0	0
Reported vaccines given not in GRITS	1 (33)	0	1 (2)
Pharmacy contacts attempted	6	63	69
No information could be provided	0	3 (5)	3 (4)
No record of vaccinations	4 (67)	60 (95)	64 (93)
Verified vaccines already in GRITS	2 (33)	0	2 (3)
Reported vaccines given not in GRITS	0	0	0
Patient/Proxy contacts attempted	7	79	86
No information could be provided	6 (86)	63 (80)	69 (80)
Not aware of vaccinations given to patient	0	2 (3)	2 (2)
Verified unvaccinated	0	14 (18)	14 (16)
Verified vaccines already in GRITS	1 (14)	0	1 (1)
Reported vaccines given not in GRITS	0	0	0
Final status after follow-up	7	79	86
No information could be provided	0	9 (11)	9 (10)
No vaccines reported	3 (43)	53 (67)	56 (65)
Verified unvaccinated	0	17 (22)	17 (20)
Verified vaccines already in GRITS	3 (43)	0	3 (4)
Reported vaccines given not in GRITS	1 (14)	0	1 (1)

Note. GRITS = Georgia Registry of Immunization Transactions and Services.

providing COVID-19 vaccine information in the 8-county Georgia COVID-NET catchment area during the study time frame, as we identified only 1 additional vaccination not in the registry and we confirmed almost one quarter of patients without a vaccine dose to be unvaccinated. A similar study in the Midwest that investigated patients without COVID-19 vaccines in IISs found that 9% reported doses when contacted and 3% had doses in PCP medical records. Although they found more doses missing from their IIS than our study did, they also had a significantly lower percentage of nonresponding patients (43% vs 80%).[12]

Our study has limitations. The COVID-NET age-stratified sample for vaccine follow-up overrepresented younger patients, which may have affected results. Additionally, our study catchment included only hospitalized patients in metro Atlanta counties and therefore may not be generalizable to other groups.

PUBLIC HEALTH IMPLICATIONS

Immunization registries are important for understanding vaccine uptake in a population, assessing vaccine effectiveness, and coordinating clinical care among providers. Accurate reporting of received vaccine doses allows researchers and clinicians to better care for their patients and communities. Pandemic era oversight encouraged providers to report COVID-19 vaccines in state IISs, likely improving their accuracy. Providers in Georgia reliably entered COVID-19 vaccine doses into GRITS from 2022 to 2023, and additional follow-up did not yield significant adjunctive information. AJPH

ABOUT THE AUTHORS

Allison D. Roebling, Nathaniel Elijah Barrera-Nitz, Kyle P. Openo, and Lucy S. Witt are with the Division of Infectious Diseases, Emory University School of Medicine, Atlanta, GA, and the Georgia

Emerging Infections Program, Atlanta. Melissa Tobin-D'Angelo is with the Georgia Department of Public Health, Atlanta, GA.

CORRESPONDENCE

Correspondence should be sent to Allison D. Roebling, Emory Health Sciences Research Building, 1760 Haygood Dr NE, 330H, Atlanta, GA 30322 (e-mail: aroebli@emory.edu). Reprints can be ordered at https://www.ajph.org by clicking the "Reprints" link.

PUBLICATION INFORMATION

Full Citation: Roebling AD, Barrera-Nitz NE, Tobin-D'Angelo M, Openo KP, Witt LS. Validating Georgia's vaccine registry for the COVID-19 2023–2024 season: true GRITS. *Am J Public Health*. 2026;116(3):368–371.

Acceptance Date: October 10, 2025.

https://doi.org/10.2105/AJPH.2025.308325

ORCID iDs:

Kyle P. Openo https://orcid.org/0009-0005-8431-6508

Lucy S. Witt https://orcid.org/0000-0003-1475-6952

CONTRIBUTORS

A. D. Roebling drafted the brief. A. D. Roebling, K. P. Openo, and L. S. Witt conceptualized and designed the work and analyzed and interpreted the data. N. E. Barrera-Nitz acquired the data. All authors revised and approved the final version of the brief to be published.

ACKNOWLEDGMENTS

The Emerging Infections Program (EIP) project described was supported by the Centers for Disease Control and Prevention (CDC; cooperative agreement NU50CK000645).

We acknowledge the work of the Georgia EIP and staff who collected and maintained these data.

Note. The contents of this article are solely the responsibility of the authors and do not necessarily represent the official views of the CDC.

CONFLICTS OF INTEREST

The authors have no conflicts of interest to disclose.

HUMAN PARTICIPANT PROTECTION

Georgia EIP surveillance activities are exempt from institutional review because it is considered public health practice at both Emory University and the Georgia Department of Public Health.

REFERENCES

1. Centers for Disease Control and Prevention. Emerging Infections Program. January 29, 2024. Available at: https://www.cdc.gov/emerging-infections-program/php/about/index.html. Accessed August 22, 2025.
2. Centers for Disease Control and Prevention. COVID-NET. June 5, 2025. Available at: https://www.cdc.gov/covid/php/covid-net/index.html. Accessed October 24, 2025.
3. Georgia Department of Public Health. Georgia Immunization Registry (GRITS). February 6, 2024. Available at: https://dph.georgia.gov/immunizations/providers-and-healthcare/georgia-immunization-registry-grits. Accessed April 4, 2025.
4. Hackell JM, Palevsky SL, Resnick M; Committee on Practice and Ambulatory Medicine, Council on Clinical Information Technology, Section on Early Career Physicians. Immunization information systems. *Pediatrics*. 2022;150(4):e2022059281. https://doi.org/10.1542/peds.2022-059281
5. Centers for Disease Control and Prevention. Initiative on immunization registries. *MMWR Morb Mortal Wkly Rep*. 2001;50(RR17):1–17. Available at: https://www.cdc.gov/mmwr/preview/mmwrhtml/rr5017a1.htm. Accessed December 2, 2025.
6. Stecher DS, Adelman R, Brinkman T, Bulloch B. Accuracy of a state immunization registry in the pediatric emergency department. *Pediatr Emerg Care*. 2008;24(2):71–74. https://doi.org/10.1097/PEC.0b013e318163db4d
7. Kolasa MS, Chilkatowsky AP, Clarke KR, Lutz JP. How complete are immunization registries? The Philadelphia story. *Ambul Pediatr*. 2006;6(1):21–24. https://doi.org/10.1016/j.ambp.2005.08.006
8. Georgia Immunization Registry Law. GA Code § 31-12-3.1 (2024).
9. Young A. Vaccine reporting spotty. *Atlanta Journal-Constitution*. October 5, 2009. Available at: https://www.ajc.com/news/local/vaccination-reporting-spotty/54v5HxTnzfpMgY0a4DxlOJ. Accessed January 24, 2025.
10. Centers for Disease Control and Prevention. CDC COVID-19 vaccination program provider requirements and support. October 6, 2023. Available at: https://www.cdc.gov/vaccines/COVID-19/vaccination-provider-support.html. Accessed January 23, 2025.
11. Surtees TC, Granade CJ, Wells C, Banks M, Lucas P, Graitcer SB. CDC COVID-19 vaccination program: healthcare provider compliance with COVID-19 vaccine requirements and recommendations. *Vaccine*. 2024;42(suppl 3):125513. https://doi.org/10.1016/j.vaccine.2023.12.023
12. McGreevy S, Murray M, Montero L, et al. Assessing the immunization information system and electronic health record interface accuracy for COVID-19 vaccinations. *JAMIA Open*. 2023;6(2):ooad026. https://doi.org/10.1093/jamiaopen/ooad026

Trends in Prepregnancy Cardiometabolic Health in Rural and Urban Areas in the United States, 2016–2023

Havisha Pedamallu, MD, MPH, Tanvi Nayak, MD, Alexa A. Freedman, PhD, Kartik K. Venkatesh, MD, PhD, William A. Grobman, MD, MBA, Sadiya S. Khan, MD, MSc, and Natalie A. Cameron, MD, MPH

Objectives. To describe differences in prepregnancy cardiometabolic health in the United States by urbanicity from 2016 to 2023.

Methods. We included 29 087 432 pregnant individuals 15 to 44 years old with data in the Centers for Disease Control and Prevention Natality Files. We calculated age-standardized trends in prepregnancy cardiometabolic health from 2016 to 2023 by urbanicity using the cardiovascular–kidney–metabolic (CKM) staging system (stage 0 [no risk factors], stage 1 [overweight/obesity], and stage 2 [diabetes or hypertension]). We used prevalence ratios to compare annual prevalence by urbanicity.

Results. From 2016 to 2023, the prevalence of prepregnancy CKM stage 0 decreased in rural and urban areas, whereas the prevalence of stages 1 and 2 increased. Specifically, stage 0 decreased from 41.5% (95% confidence interval [CI] = 41.4%, 41.7%) to 35.6% (95% CI = 35.4%, 35.7%) in rural areas and from 48.2% (95% CI = 48.1%, 48.3%) to 40.7% (95% CI = 40.6%, 40.7%) in urban areas. Prevalence ratios for stages 0 through 2 in 2016 were 0.86 (95% CI = 0.86, 0.87), 1.12 (95% CI = 1.11, 1.12), and 1.36 (95% CI = 1.34, 1.39), respectively, in rural relative to urban areas and remained stable over the study period.

Conclusions. In this national sample, prepregnancy cardiometabolic health decreased from 2016 to 2023 in urban and rural communities and exhibited a persistent gap, with rural areas more severely affected. (*Am J Public Health*. 2026;116(3):372–375. https://doi.org/10.2105/AJPH.2025.308299)

AJPH March 2026, Vol. 116, No. 3

Maternal health in the United States has decreased in recent years, disproportionately affecting women in rural areas.[1–3] In comparison with urban areas, rates of maternal complications in rural areas are approximately 10% higher for new-onset hypertensive disorders of pregnancy, 20% higher for gestational diabetes, and nearly double for maternal mortality.[1,3,4] Poor prepregnancy cardiometabolic health contributes to hypertensive disorders of pregnancy, gestational diabetes, congenital abnormalities, maternal intensive care unit admissions, preterm birth, low birth weight, and fetal death.[5]

The American Heart Association's cardiovascular–kidney–metabolic (CKM) construct integrates interconnected risk factors, staging progression from ideal health (stage 0) to excess adiposity (stage 1), cardiovascular disease (CVD) risk factors (e.g., hypertension; stage 2), subclinical CVD (stage 3), and overt CVD (stage 4).[6] Women in rural areas have been shown to have a higher prevalence of individual prepregnancy cardiometabolic risk factors, but contemporary data regarding the cumulative burden of these risk factors are lacking.[4,7] In this study, we used the CKM construct to describe trends in prepregnancy cardiometabolic health in the United States by urbanicity from 2016 to 2023.

METHODS

We conducted a serial cross-sectional analysis of all US live births from 2016 to 2023 in the Centers for Disease Control and Prevention Natality Database. Data were drawn from birth certificates and standardized maternal and facility worksheets. We included births to people 15 to 44 years of age and excluded records missing data on prepregnancy body mass index, diabetes, and hypertension.

The primary outcome was prepregnancy cardiometabolic health, defined according to the CKM staging system (stage 0 [no overweight/obesity, diabetes, or hypertension], stage 1 [overweight/obesity only], and stage 2 [diabetes or hypertension]). Overweight/obesity was defined as a body mass index of 25.0 kg/m^2 or higher. Subclinical CVD (CKM stage 3) and CVD (CKM stage 4) were not reported in this database.

We calculated the age-standardized annual prevalence of each CKM stage (standardized to the 2016 birthing population) and classified births as occurring in rural or urban areas using the 2013 National Center for Health Statistics Urban-Rural Scheme for Counties.[8] In this classification scheme, urban areas include large, medium, and small metropolitan areas and large fringe areas. We calculated age-standardized prevalence ratios (PRs) to compare the prevalence of CKM stages by urbanicity and calculated the average annual percentage change (AAPC) to assess trends. We conducted a sensitivity analysis limited to births among nulliparous individuals to ensure that our findings were not influenced by outcomes from repeat pregnancies. We used Stata SE version 14.2 (StataCorp LP, College Station, TX) and Joinpoint (Surveillance Research Program, National Cancer Institute, Bethesda, MD) software in conducting our analyses.

RESULTS

Of the 29 087 432 included births, 86.4% of the birthing people lived in urban areas and 13.6% lived in rural areas; 0.7% identified as American Indian or Alaska Native, 6.2% as Asian, 24.1% as Hispanic, 2.3% as multiracial, 0.3% as Native Hawaiian or Pacific Islander, 14.2% as non-Hispanic Black or African American, and 51.4% as non-Hispanic White. Individuals with live births in rural areas were more likely to be younger than 25 years (33.0% vs 21.6%; $P < .001$) and to identify as non-Hispanic White (72.1% vs 48.2%; $P < .001$).

The prevalence of prepregnancy CKM stage 0 was lower in rural than urban areas in each year from 2016 to 2023 (Figure 1). In rural areas, the prevalence of CKM stage 0 decreased from 41.5% (95% confidence interval [CI] = 41.4%, 41.7%) to 35.6% (35.4%, 35.7%; AAPC = −2.3% per year; 95% CI = −2.7%, −2.0%). A similar decrease was observed in urban areas for CKM stage 0, from 48.2% (95% CI = 48.1%, 48.3%) to 40.7% (95% CI = 40.6%, 40.7%; AAPC = −2.5% per year; 95% CI = −2.7%, −2.3%). Prevalence ratios comparing the prevalence of CKM stage 0 in rural and urban areas were stable from 2016 (adjusted PR [APR] = 0.86; 95% CI = 0.86, 0.87) to 2023 (0.87; 95% CI = 0.87, 0.88).

From 2016 to 2023, the prevalence of prepregnancy CKM stage 1 and stage 2 was higher in rural than urban areas. The prevalence of CKM stage 1 increased from 55.3% (95% CI = 55.1%, 55.5%) to 59.4% (95% CI = 59.2, 59.6; AAPC = 1.1% per year; 95% CI = 0.8%, 1.4%) in rural areas and from 49.5% (95% CI = 49.4%, 49.5%) to 55.6% (95% CI = 55.5%, 55.6%; AAPC = 1.7% per year; 95% CI = 1.5%, 2.0%) in urban areas (2016 APR = 1.12; 95% CI = 1.11, 1.12; 2023 APR = 1.07; 95% CI = 1.06, 1.07). For CKM stage 2, the prevalence increased from 3.2% (95% CI = 3.1%, 3.2%) to 5.0% (95% CI = 5.0%, 5.1%; AAPC = 6.8% per year; 95% CI = 6.4%, 7.3%) in rural areas and from 2.3% (95% CI = 2.3%, 2.4%) to 3.8% (95% CI = 3.8%, 3.8%; AAPC = 7.2% per year; 95% CI = 6.6%, 7.7%) in urban areas. Prevalence ratios comparing the prevalence of CKM stage 2 in rural and urban areas were stable from 2016 to 2023 (2016 APR = 1.36; 95% CI = 1.34, 1.39; 2023 APR = 1.33; 95% CI = 1.31, 1.35).

Patterns were overall similar in a sensitivity analysis of births to nulliparous individuals.

DISCUSSION

In this national sample of US live births from 2016 to 2023, prepregnancy cardiometabolic health, as measured via CKM staging, decreased with a persistent rural–urban gap. By 2023, 40% or fewer of individuals in either setting entered pregnancy with ideal cardiometabolic health (CKM stage 0). The prevalence of CKM stage 2 (diabetes or hypertension) increased consistently and remained 30% higher in rural areas.

This study builds on existing literature by applying the American Heart Association's CKM framework to prepregnancy health, offering a multisystem view of risk.[4,6,7] We demonstrated rapidly accelerating rates of prepregnancy CKM stage 2 with a persistent rural–urban gap. Although our data cannot directly assess drivers of worsening CKM health, likely contributors

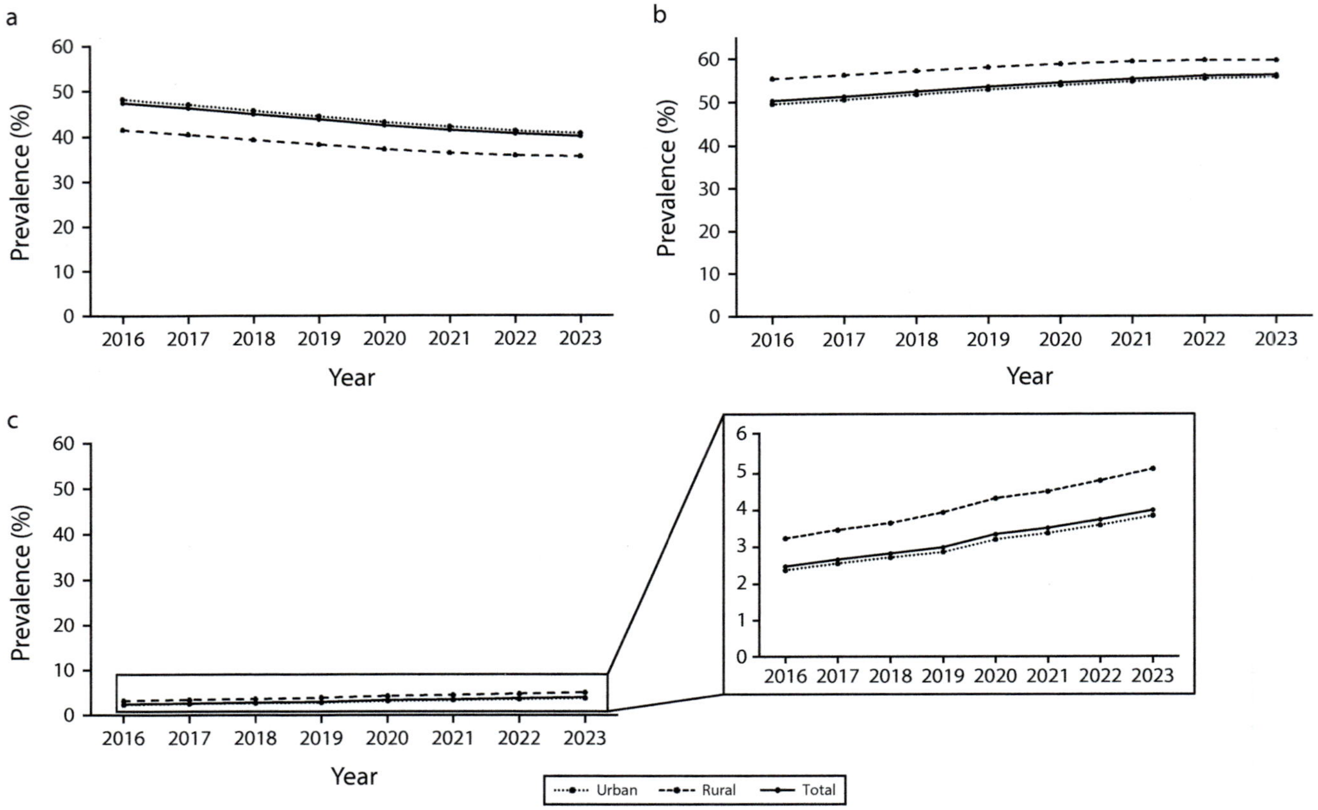

FIGURE 1— Age-Adjusted Prevalence of Prepregnancy CKM Syndrome Stages 0 (A), 1 (B), and 2 (C): United States, 2016–2023

Note. Cardiovascular–kidney–metabolic (CKM) syndrome stage definitions are as follows: stage 0 = no prepregnancy overweight/obesity, diabetes, or hypertension; stage 1 = prepregnancy overweight/obesity without diabetes or hypertension; stage 2 = prepregnancy diabetes or hypertension.

include limited access to preventive care and unmet social needs (e.g., food insecurity, walkability).[9] These barriers are often exacerbated in rural areas by physician shortages, fewer prenatal care services, long travel distances, and limited resources for health departments.[3]

This study has several limitations. First, the data set includes only live births, excluding pregnancies ending in miscarriage, stillbirth, or termination, which may underestimate poor prepregnancy cardiometabolic health. Second, type of diabetes is not specified on birth certificates. However, because both type 1 and type 2 diabetes are classified as CKM stage 2, this does not affect our results. Third, the absence of laboratory values, kidney function data, and CVD information likely led to overestimation of ideal health (CKM stage 0) and underestimation of stage 2.

Fourth, data were not available on measures of body composition other than body mass index (e.g., waist circumference) to confirm diagnoses of excess adiposity as now recommended by the Lancet Commission on Clinical Obesity.[10] Fifth, some degree of misclassification of obesity, diabetes, and hypertension is possible, although these variables are collected via standardized protocols and are comparable across birth certificate revisions. Finally, underreporting may be more pronounced in rural areas as a result of limited care access and diagnostic testing. Thus, we may have underestimated rural–urban differences in this study.

PUBLIC HEALTH IMPLICATIONS

Rural areas bear a disproportionate burden of stage 2 CKM, underscoring the need for urgent public health efforts to improve prepregnancy CKM health and reduce maternal disparities. The American Heart Association's presidential advisory on rural health recommends reforms such as community-based rural clinician training programs, expanded school-based health centers, improved telehealth access and infrastructure, and Medicaid expansion.[3] Specifically, Medicaid expansion and insurance market reform may help improve health and reduce chronic disease mortality in rural areas, particularly in states with lower expansion rates.[3] Past studies have linked Medicaid expansion to increased use of diabetes and cardiovascular medications and improved health care access among individuals of reproductive age with the lowest coverage levels.[11,12] More research is needed to better understand how Medicaid expansion and other public health efforts can reduce rural–urban disparities and mitigate decreasing prepregnancy CKM health. AJPH

ABOUT THE AUTHORS

At the time of this study, Havisha Pedamallu and Tanvi Nayak were with the Feinberg School of Medicine, Northwestern University, Chicago, IL. Alexa A. Freedman is with the Department of Preventive Medicine, Division of Epidemiology, Feinberg School of Medicine, Northwestern University. Kartik K. Venkatesh is with the Department of Obstetrics and Gynecology, The Ohio State University College of Medicine, Columbus. William A. Grobman is with the Department of Obstetrics and Gynecology, Warren Alpert Medical School, Brown University, Providence, RI. Sadiya S. Khan is with the Department of Medicine, Division of Cardiology, and the Department of Preventive Medicine, Division of Epidemiology, Feinberg School of Medicine, Northwestern University. Natalie A. Cameron is with the Department of Medicine, Division of General Internal Medicine, and the Department of Preventive Medicine, Division of Epidemiology, Feinberg School of Medicine, Northwestern University.

CORRESPONDENCE

Correspondence should be sent to Natalie A. Cameron, MD, MPH, Department of Medicine (Division of General Internal Medicine), Department of Preventive Medicine (Epidemiology), Northwestern University Feinberg School of Medicine, 750 N Lake Shore Dr, Floor 10, Chicago, IL 60611 (e-mail: natalie.cameron@northwestern.edu). Reprints can be ordered at https://www.ajph.org by clicking the "Reprints" link.

PUBLICATION INFORMATION

Full Citation: Pedamallu H, Nayak T, Freedman AA, et al. Trends in prepregnancy cardiometabolic health in rural and urban areas in the United States, 2016–2023. *Am J Public Health*. 2026;116(3):372–375.

Acceptance Date: September 14, 2025.

DOI: https://doi.org/10.2105/AJPH.2025.308299

ORCID iDs:

Havisha Pedamallu https://orcid.org/0000-0002-1753-1153

Alexa A. Freedman https://orcid.org/0000-0001-9745-7768

Natalie A. Cameron https://orcid.org/0000-0002-0613-7580

CONTRIBUTORS

H. Pedamallu contributed to conception, data analysis, and writing. T. Nayak, A. A. Freedman, K. K. Venkatesh, W. A. Grobman, and S. S. Khan contributed to critical review and editing. N. A. Cameron contributed to conceptualization, methodology, supervision, and reviewing and editing.

ACKNOWLEDGMENTS

Natalie A. Cameron received funding from the American Heart Association (grant 25CDA1449707).

CONFLICTS OF INTEREST

The authors have no conflicts of interest.

HUMAN PARTICIPANT PROTECTION

This study was exempt from institutional review board approval because publicly available, deidentified data were used.

REFERENCES

1. Cameron NA, Everitt I, Seegmiller LE, Yee LM, Grobman WA, Khan SS. Trends in the incidence of new-onset hypertensive disorders of pregnancy among rural and urban areas in the United States, 2007 to 2019. *J Am Heart Assoc.* 2022; 11(2):e023791. https://doi.org/10.1161/JAHA.121.023791
2. Freaney PM, Harrington K, Molsberry R, et al. Temporal trends in adverse pregnancy outcomes in birthing individuals aged 15 to 44 years in the United States, 2007 to 2019. *J Am Heart Assoc.* 2022;11(11):e025050. https://doi.org/10.1161/JAHA.121.025050
3. Harrington RA, Califf RM, Balamurugan A, et al. Call to action: rural health: a presidential advisory from the American Heart Association and American Stroke Association. *Circulation.* 2020;141(10): e615–e644. https://doi.org/10.1161/CIR.0000000000000753
4. Venkatesh KK, Huang X, Cameron NA, et al. Rural-urban disparities in pregestational and gestational diabetes in pregnancy: serial, cross-sectional analysis of over 12 million pregnancies. *BJOG.* 2024;131(1):26–35. https://doi.org/10.1111/1471-0528.17587
5. Khan SS, Brewer LC, Canobbio MM, et al. Optimizing prepregnancy cardiovascular health to improve outcomes in pregnant and postpartum individuals and offspring: a scientific statement from the American Heart Association. *Circulation.* 2023;147(7):e76–e91. https://doi.org/10.1161/CIR.0000000000001124
6. Ndumele CE, Rangaswami J, Chow SL, et al. Cardiovascular-kidney-metabolic health: a presidential advisory from the American Heart Association. *Circulation.* 2023;148(20):1606–1635. https://doi.org/10.1161/CIR.0000000000001184
7. Cameron NA, Molsberry R, Pierce JB, et al. Pre-pregnancy hypertension among women in rural and urban areas of the United States. *J Am Coll Cardiol.* 2020;76(22):2611–2619. https://doi.org/10.1016/j.jacc.2020.09.601
8. Ingram DD, Franco SJ. 2013 NCHS urban-rural classification scheme for counties. *Vital Health Stat 2.* 2014(166):1–73. Available at: https://www.cdc.gov/nchs/data/series/sr_02/sr02_166.pdf. Accessed October 21, 2025.
9. Powell-Wiley TM, Baumer Y, Baah FO, et al. Social determinants of cardiovascular disease. *Circ Res.* 2022;130(5):782–799. https://doi.org/10.1161/CIRCRESAHA.121.319811
10. Rubino F, Cummings DE, Eckel RH, et al. Definition and diagnostic criteria of clinical obesity. *Lancet Diabetes Endocrinol.* 2025;13(3):221–262. https://doi.org/10.1016/S2213-8587(24)00316-4
11. Ghosh A, Simon K, Sommers BD. The effect of health insurance on prescription drug use among low-income adults: evidence from recent Medicaid expansions. *J Health Econ.* 2019;63: 64–80. https://doi.org/10.1016/j.jhealeco.2018.11.002
12. Margerison CE, MacCallum CL, Chen J, Zamani-Hank Y, Kaestner R. Impacts of Medicaid expansion on health among women of reproductive age. *Am J Prev Med.* 2020;58(1):1–11. https://doi.org/10.1016/j.amepre.2019.08.019

Estimated Number of People Who Inject Drugs in the United States, 2022

Heather Bradley, PhD, MHS, Sara N. Glick, PhD, MPH, and Eric W. Hall, PhD, MPH

Objectives. To estimate the population size of people who inject drugs (PWID) in the United States in 2022.

Methods. We constructed a hybrid estimator, which applied the ratio of nonfatal to fatal overdose among PWID to convert estimated injection-involved overdose deaths to the number of nonfatal overdoses. We divided the number of nonfatal overdose events by the prevalence of nonfatal overdose to generate PWID population size estimates.

Results. There were an estimated 2 392 100 (95% confidence interval = 1 323 300, 4 648 100) PWID in 2022, which was 35% lower than the 2018 estimate. Most PWID were male and non-Hispanic White. The US South had the highest number of PWID.

Conclusions. Reduced PWID population size may reflect improved data inputs or a true decline in the number of PWID because of high levels of overdose fatality or shifts in routes of drug consumption. These data are essential for determining needs for prevention services and rates of morbidity and mortality among PWID. (*Am J Public Health*. 2026;116(3):376–379. https://doi.org/10.2105/AJPH.2025.308310)

AJPH March 2026, Vol. 116, No. 3

The use of injectable drugs has increased as a result of the US opioid crisis.[1] Injection drug use (IDU) carries infectious disease risk for people who inject drugs (PWID).[2] Moreover, the drug supply has become more lethal, leading to increased overdose.[1] Although surveillance data can be used to identify trends in adverse health events among PWID (e.g., HIV infection, overdose), it is difficult to determine to what extent changes in these health outcomes result from changes in PWID population size, increased lethality of the drug supply, or changes in injection behaviors. The answer to this question requires, in part, a routinely updated estimate of PWID population size.

Previous research estimated that there were 3.7 million PWID in the United States during 2018, a 3- to 5-fold increase from 2011.[3] However, substance use patterns are highly dynamic, and it is critical to routinely estimate PWID population size. For example, data from after 2018 indicate shifts from injection to smoking of fentanyl.[4,5] Data-driven resource allocation and monitoring for interventions aiming to reduce morbidity and mortality among PWID depend on routinely updated prevalence estimates. We replicated methodology employed for a previously published 2018 PWID population size estimate using the most recently available surveillance data inputs and generated a PWID population size estimate for 2022.

METHODS

We used a hybrid estimator for PWID population size using a combination of surveillance and research data. Our methods replicated those used for a 2018 estimate,[3] and full methodological details are included in the supplemental material (available as a supplement to the online version of this article at http://www.ajph.org). Briefly, we used a modified multiplier approach in a stepwise fashion (Figure A, available as a supplement to the online version of this article at http://www.ajph.org).

First, we estimated the number of injection-involved overdose deaths in 2022 based on the likelihood of injection for substances involved in all overdose deaths recorded in the National Vital Statistics System.[6] Second, we estimated the number of nonfatal overdose events among PWID by multiplying the number of injection-involved overdose deaths by a ratio of nonfatal to fatal overdose among PWID (16.6; 95% confidence interval [CI] = 9.2, 30.3). We derived this ratio from a meta-analysis of published US research studies with data collected between 2016 and 2023.[7] Finally, we estimated the total number of PWID by dividing the number of nonfatal overdose events in the previous step by the percentage of PWID who experienced a nonfatal overdose during 2022 using National HIV Behavioral Surveillance System data.[8]

When possible, we conducted this analysis within strata defined by sex, age group, race/ethnicity, and US Census region. To quantify uncertainty, we defined distributions around each input and used Monte Carlo simulation (k = 10 000) to resample from each distribution. The median defined our point estimates, and the 2.5th and 97.5th percentiles of the resulting distributions constituted the 95% CIs. We computed IDU prevalence by dividing estimated population size by 2022 adult population size for each strata.[9] Lastly, we conducted a sensitivity analysis varying the nonfatal to fatal overdose ratio from 5 to 40, which encompasses the meta-analyzed estimate's CI. We conducted statistical analyses using R version 4.4.2 (R Core Team, Vienna, Austria).

RESULTS

An estimated 2 392 100 people (95% CI = 1 323 300, 4 648 100) injected drugs in the United States in 2022, corresponding to 0.9% (95% CI = 0.5%, 1.8%) of the adult population (Table 1). The 2022 PWID population size estimate and corresponding prevalence estimate are 35.3% and 37.2% lower, respectively, than previously estimated for 2018.[3] Sensitivity analyses showed

TABLE 1— Estimated Number of Adults Who Inject Drugs: United States, 2022

	Overdose Deaths, No.	Adult Population in 2022,[9] No.	Injection-Involved Overdose Deaths, No. (95% CI)	Nonfatal Overdose Events, No. (95% CI)	Population Size of People Who Inject Drugs	
					No. (95% CI)	% (95% CI)
Overall	106 928	260 836 730	42 190 (41 989, 42 382)	704 300 (389 400, 1 286 500)	2 392 100 (1 323 300, 4 648 100)	0.92 (0.51, 1.78)
US Census region						
Northeast	20 422	45 544 589	8 029 (7 982, 8 074)	134 100 (74 000, 244 700)	458 200 (253 200, 838 000)	1.01 (0.56, 1.84)
Midwest	21 498	53 626 659	8 675 (8 596, 8 757)	144 800 (80 000, 264 900)	481 900 (265 000, 881 100)	0.90 (0.49, 1.64)
South	41 881	100 098 310	17 311 (17 156, 17 464)	289 100 (159 800, 527 400)	979 300 (541 300, 1 786 000)	0.98 (0.54, 1.78)
West	23 127	61 567 172	8 175 (8 093, 8 258)	136 400 (75 400, 249 300)	469 700 (259 400, 862 600)	0.76 (0.42, 1.40)
Sex						
Male	75 234	128 209 284	30 582 (30 407, 30 754)	510 600 (282 100, 932 100)	1 701 600 (943 200, 3 106 900)	1.33 (0.74, 2.42)
Female	31 694	132 627 446	11 606 (11 514, 11 702)	193 600 (107 100, 353 800)	686 300 (378 500, 1 257 000)	0.52 (0.29, 0.95)
Race/ethnicity						
Hispanic	13 874	44 856 597	5 594 (5 530, 5 657)	93 400 (51 600, 170 700)	348 000 (191 800, 636 600)	0.78 (0.43, 1.42)
Non-Hispanic White single-race	68 126	160 857 594	31 457 (31 293, 31 618)	525 000 (290 300, 959 500)	1 724 800 (955 200, 3 136 900)	1.07 (0.59, 1.95)
Non-Hispanic Black single-race	20 729	31 999 309	3 636 (3 551, 3 721)	60 800 (33 500, 111 100)	243 100 (134 500, 445 200)	0.76 (0.42, 1.39)
Non-Hispanic other/multirace	4 199	23 123 230	1 503 (1 472, 1 533)	25 100 (13 800, 45 900)	73 600 (40 300, 135 700)	0.32 (0.17, 0.59)
Age, y						
18–39	43 181	99 097 380	20 174 (20 058, 20 291)	337 000 (186 300, 615 000)	1 004 000 (556 900, 1 834 900)	1.01 (0.56, 1.85)
≥40	63 747	161 739 350	22 013 (21 853, 22 173)	367 500 (203 000, 671 900)	1 387 000 (766 200, 2 521 100)	0.86 (0.47, 1.56)

Note. CI = confidence interval.

that population size estimates stayed within the CI when the nonfatal to fatal overdose ratio was held within its CI range (9.2, 30.3; Figure B [available as a supplement to the online version of this article at http://www.ajph.org]). In 2022, most PWID were male (71.1%) and non-Hispanic White (72.1%). The US South had the highest estimated number of PWID by geography (979 300; 95% CI = 541 300, 1 786 000). Although an estimated 58% of PWID were aged 40 years or older, IDU prevalence was similar (1.01%; 95% CI = 0.56%, 1.85%) among persons aged 18 to 39 years compared with those aged 40 years or older (0.86%; 95% CI = 0.47%, 1.56%).

DISCUSSION

Overall, we estimated approximately 35% fewer PWID in 2022 than the 2018 estimate. This reduction is likely attributable to an important difference in model inputs but also to real demographic and behavioral changes among PWID. In terms of model inputs, the ratio of nonfatal to fatal overdose among PWID, which we used to convert estimated injection-involved overdose deaths to the number of nonfatal overdoses, was 16.6 in this analysis and 40.5 in the 2018 analysis.[7] Both ratios were derived from meta-analyses, but we derived the ratio used for our 2022 estimate from more current, US-specific estimates, whereas the previous ratio was derived from older estimates from Organisation for Economic Co-operation and Development countries.

Observed changes in the PWID population may have also resulted in a real reduction in IDU prevalence. First, as the drug supply became more lethal during this time,[1] overdose mortality rates among PWID increased alongside observed increases among other people who use drugs.[1] The estimated number of injection-involved deaths was 49% greater in 2022 than in 2018,[3] whereas the percentage of PWID experiencing nonfatal overdose annually was nearly the same in each year (~28%).[8,10] Second, there is evidence indicating transitions from injection to smoking as a primary mode of substance administration for some opioids.[4,5] Third, the COVID-19 pandemic caused substantially higher mortality rates in 2022 than in 2018 among the general population, and PWID may have experienced elevated COVID-19–related mortality risk because of high prevalence of homelessness and low prevalence of clinical care receipt.[2]

Population sizes and prevalence estimates have distinct implications for policies and interventions. Estimated population sizes indicate the overall magnitude of groups in need of services, whereas prevalence estimates indicate risk across population groups and disparities in service needs. Here, we observed large differences in the population sizes of PWID by racial/ethnic groups but much smaller differences in prevalence across these groups. Surveillance data indicate large increases in overdose mortality among Black communities and other minoritized populations and underscore this finding.[11] From a health equity perspective, substance use prevention, harm reduction, and treatment services for minoritized racial/ethnic groups are urgently needed.

The primary limitation of our approach was its dependence on an estimate of the nonfatal to fatal overdose ratio, which we derived from meta-analysis because of lack of otherwise available data. Heterogeneity across meta-analyzed rates of nonfatal and fatal overdose resulted in imprecision of the ratio. We quantified this imprecision in 95% CIs of the population size estimates, and this input contributed most of the uncertainty we observed in the estimates. Additionally, although the updated estimates reflect a more accurate and current ratio of nonfatal to fatal overdose than used for the 2018 estimates,[3] future estimates would benefit greatly from ratios that are specific to region and demographic groups.

PUBLIC HEALTH IMPLICATIONS

The estimated number of PWID declined from 2018 to 2022. Much of this decline is likely attributable to increased overdose mortality and improvements in model inputs. However, there is also a growing literature base demonstrating transitions from injection to smoking among some people who use drugs.[4,5] When feasible, harm reduction organizations such as syringe service programs are responding to these dynamics by shifting their services to provide safer smoking supplies, and these efforts should be supported by both accommodating policies and increased resource allocation. Smoking carries less infectious disease and possibly less overdose risk than injection,[12] but communities will need to monitor potential increases in overdose risk from fentanyl smoking among new users. Continuing to expand access to harm reduction and other health services is an urgent need for PWID.

It is important to continue to monitor PWID population size over time, across geographies, and by demographic characteristics. PWID denominators allow risk for overdose and infectious diseases to be expressed per population rates. Without denominators, changing numbers of adverse events do not tell us the extent to which IDU prevalence is changing versus the extent to which risk environments, behaviors, or substance lethality are changing. Developing and implementing effective strategies for improving the health of PWID depends on understanding how each of these factors influence trends in health outcomes over time. AJPH

ABOUT THE AUTHORS

Heather Bradley is with Emory University Rollins School of Public Health, Atlanta, GA. Sara N. Glick is with the School of Medicine, University of Washington, Seattle, and Public Health–Seattle & King County, Seattle, WA. Eric W. Hall is with the Oregon Health & Science University–Portland State University, School of Public Health, Portland.

CORRESPONDENCE

Correspondence should be sent to Heather Bradley, PhD, 1518 Clifton Rd NE, Atlanta, GA 30322 (e-mail: hbradl2@emory.edu). Reprints can be ordered at https://www.ajph.org by clicking the "Reprints" link.

PUBLICATION INFORMATION

Full Citation: Bradley H, Glick SN, Hall EW. Estimated number of people who inject drugs in the United States, 2022. *Am J Public Health.* 2026;116(3):376–379.

Acceptance Date: October 1, 2025.

DOI: https://doi.org/10.2105/AJPH.2025.308310

ORCID iDs:

Heather Bradley https://orcid.org/0000-0002-7667-4197

Eric W. Hall https://orcid.org/0000-0003-0244-7458

CONTRIBUTORS

H. Bradley and E. W. Hall conceptualized and designed the work and acquired, analyzed, and interpreted the data. S. N. Glick made substantial contributions to data interpretation. All authors drafted the article, revised it critically for important intellectual content, and approved the version to be published.

ACKNOWLEDGMENTS

This work was supported by the Centers for Disease Control and Prevention (CDC), National Center for HIV, Viral Hepatitis, STD, and Tuberculosis Prevention (grant U38PS004650) and the National Institutes of Health (NIH), National Institute on Drug Abuse (grant R01DA051302).

The authors are grateful to scientists at the CDC, Divisions of HIV Prevention and Viral Hepatitis for their assistance with this work.

Note. The contents of this article are solely the responsibility of the authors and do not necessarily represent the official views of the NIH or the CDC.

CONFLICTS OF INTEREST

S. N. Glick has received funding from Cepheid for research unrelated to this work. H. Bradley and E. W. Hall have no conflicts of interest to disclose.

HUMAN PARTICIPANT PROTECTION

This work is a secondary analysis of publicly available and de-identified data sets and so was exempt from institutional review board review.

REFERENCES

1. Garnett MF, Miniño AM. Drug overdose deaths in the United States, 2003–2023. *NCHS Data Brief.* No. 522. National Center for Health Statistics; 2024. Available at: https://www.cdc.gov/nchs/data/databriefs/db522.pdf. Accessed November 21, 2025.
2. Centers for Disease Control and Prevention. HIV infection and HIV-associated behaviors among persons who inject drugs—23 metropolitan statistical areas, United States, 2018. *MMWR Morb Mortal Wkly Rep.* 2021;70(42):1459–1465. https://doi.org/10.15585/mmwr.mm7042a1
3. Bradley H, Hall EW, Asher A, et al. Estimated number of people who inject drugs in the United States. *Clin Infect Dis.* 2023;76(1):96–102. https://doi.org/10.1093/cid/ciac543
4. Kral AH, Lambdin BH, Browne EN, et al. Transition from injecting opioids to smoking fentanyl in San Francisco, California. *Drug Alcohol Depend.* 2021;227:109003. https://doi.org/10.1016/j.drugalcdep.2021.109003
5. Centers for Disease Control and Prevention. Routes of drug use among drug overdose deaths—United States, 2020–2022. *MMWR Morb Mortal Wkly Rep.* 2024;73(6):124–130. https://doi.org/10.15585/mmwr.mm7306a2
6. National Center for Health Statistics. Mortality data on CDC WONDER. November 20, 2025. Available at: https://wonder.cdc.gov/mcd.html. Accessed November 21, 2025.
7. Shealey J, Hall EW, Pigott TD, et al. Systematic review and meta-analysis to estimate the burden of non-fatal and fatal overdose among people who inject drugs living in the US and comparator countries: 2010–2023. *medRxiv.* [Preprint August 2024]. https://doi.org/10.1101/2024.08.14.24310813. Available at: https://www.medrxiv.org/content/10.1101/2024.08.14.24310813v1. Accessed November 21, 2025.
8. Centers for Disease Control and Prevention. HIV infection risk, prevention, and testing behaviors among persons who inject drugs national HIV behavioral surveillance, 20 US cities. February 1, 2024. HIV Surveillance Special Report No. 35. 2024. Available at: https://stacks.cdc.gov/view/cdc/150464. Accessed November 21, 2025.
9. Centers for Disease Control and Prevention. Single-race population estimates. Available at: https://wonder.cdc.gov/single-race-population.html. Accessed February 14, 2025.
10. Centers for Disease Control and Prevention. HIV infection risk, prevention, and testing behaviors among persons who inject drugs—National HIV Behavioral Surveillance: injection drug use, 23 US cities, 2018. HIV Surveillance Special Report No. 24. February 2020. Available at: https://stacks.cdc.gov/view/cdc/106349. Accessed November 21, 2025.
11. Smith MK, Planalp C, Bennis SL, et al. Widening racial disparities in the US overdose epidemic. *Am J Prev Med.* 2025;68(4):745–753. https://doi.org/10.1016/j.amepre.2024.12.020
12. Megerian CE, Bair L, Smith J, et al. Health risks associated with smoking versus injecting fentanyl among people who use drugs in California. *Drug Alcohol Depend.* 2024;255(111053):111053. https://doi.org/10.1016/j.drugalcdep.2023.111053

Racial Disparities in Victim Compensation Program Claim Approvals for Adult Survivors of Sexual Assault: 18 US States, 2015–2023

Samuel Dickman, MD, Jeremy Levine, PhD, Chalem Bolton, PhD, Anna Conway, BA, and Kelly Russell, PhD

Objectives. To examine racial/ethnic disparities in victim compensation claim approval rates for adult survivors of sexual assault.

Methods. We analyzed administrative data from 18 US state victim compensation programs (2015–2023), covering 45 934 claims from adult sexual assault survivors. We used multivariable linear probability models to examine predictors of claim approval, adjusting for survivor age and state and year fixed effects.

Results. Of all claims, 93.4% were from women; 41.7% were from White, 20.8% were from Latina, and 15% were from Black applicants. Black and Indigenous women's claims were less likely to be approved than were White women's ($P < .001$). The most common denial reason was lack of evidence that a crime had occurred (34.4%). Racial/ethnic disparities appear to be driven by administrative paperwork burdens. Approval rates varied widely, from 29.4% in Illinois to 94.1% in New Hampshire. Claims referred by hospitals or law enforcement had higher probabilities of approval than did those referred by other sources.

Conclusions. Racial disparities exist in victim compensation claim approvals.

Public Health Implications. Removing police reporting requirements and simplifying application processes could reduce racial disparities in access to compensation for survivors of sexual assault.
(*Am J Public Health.* 2026;116(3):380–386. https://doi.org/10.2105/AJPH.2025.308304)

AJPH March 2026, Vol. 116, No. 3

One in 4 women is raped and 54.3% of women and 30.7% of men experience other forms of sexual violence during their lifetimes.[1] Most survivors of sexual assault require acute and long-term physical and mental health care services, as well as forensic medical examinations. Yet many survivors of sexual assault are uninsured,[2] and even those with private insurance coverage often face large out-of-pocket costs.[3] Such financial barriers may discourage care seeking and contribute to low reporting rates.[4]

State-administered crime victim compensation programs aim to alleviate survivors' financial burdens by covering costs associated with violent crimes, including medical expenses, mental health counseling, forensic medical examinations, and some other expenses (e.g., relocation). Most funds for sexual assault survivors are used for health-related services.[5] Victim compensation can be accessed only after other resources (e.g., insurance and civil judgments) have been exhausted. Claims are processed outside the criminal justice system and do not require an offender to be charged or convicted.[6] By law, the objective severity of injury should have no bearing on the decision to approve a claim. The 3 key eligibility requirements are that claimants be survivors of crime, be innocent (i.e., they were not committing a crime during their victimization and did not engage in behavior that may have contributed to the crime), and have out-of-pocket expenses.

Women of color are disproportionately affected by sexual violence[7] and may face additional barriers in accessing public victim compensation programs. The case-by-case nature of approvals introduces potential for racially discriminatory compensation determinations[8]; for example, state laws require police to verify that claimants were survivors of crime, were cooperative, and did not engage in conduct that may have directly or indirectly led to their victimization (which is rare among sexual assault claimants).[9] This can create a racialized organizational process if, for instance, people of color are less likely to cooperate with police or the police are less likely to recognize survivors' trauma.

We used novel administrative data obtained through freedom of information requests to examine patterns of victim compensation program claims, denial rates, and racial/ethnic disparities in approval rates for adult survivors of sexual assault.

METHODS

We obtained individual claim-level data on victim compensation requests and decisions on awards and denials from 18 US states, covering the period 2015 to 2023 (Table A [available as a supplement to the online version of this article at http://www.ajph.org] details geographic and temporal coverage). First, we sought these data by e-mailing the person of contact, who submitted the annual performance report to the federal Office for Victims of Crime for all 50 states. Eleven states responded and provided data either immediately or following a brief conversation with a member of the research team. We obtained data from 6 additional states from formal freedom of information requests. Data from 1 state, Oklahoma, was published online by a journalist investigating the program.[10] Four states provided aggregated data or data that were unusable because of missing information. The remaining states ignored the team's initial e-mail and subsequent follow-up messages and either denied or did not respond to formal freedom of information requests.

The data included survivor race, gender, and age; crime type; application year; decision on claim; and denial reason, if applicable. Massachusetts did not provide age information, and the age categories supplied by California and by New York were incompatible owing to overlapping age bands. Four states (Arizona, Minnesota, Oklahoma, and Texas) provided data on referral sources. Seven states organized data by claimant, with a variable indicating the claimant's relationship to the survivor. To properly interpret demographic variables across states, we limited our analysis to claimants who submitted claims on behalf of themselves from these states.

We hand coded each claim from adult sexual assault survivors to determine approvals and denial reasons. Four states (Florida, Illinois, Minnesota, and Texas) reported conflicting approval and denial information for some claims (e.g., indicated some claims were both approved and denied); we coded these as approved if any payment to the claimant above $0 was reported. Six states allow multiple denial reasons per claim. Five of those states (Florida, Minnesota, New Hampshire, Rhode Island, and Washington) listed reasons in a sequential list, and we used the first reason listed. California indicated each denial reason in separate columns. In analyses of approval rates, we included all approved and denied claims from California to ensure accurate comparisons across states. In analyses of denial rates, however, we limited data from California to claims with a single denial reason to avoid overweighting claims from California.

We limited our analysis to sexual assault claims by women that resulted in victim compensation decisions, excluding duplicates and withdrawn claims. Data from New York were limited to adults aged 20 and older because of data availability.

Our analysis unfolded in 3 parts. First, we analyzed approvals. We tabulated compensation claims and approval rates for women sexual assault survivors by race/ethnicity and age for the 18 states. We then fit a linear probability model (results of which are nearly identical to models using logistic regression methods)[11] to examine racial/ethnic differences in claim approval, with approval coded as a binary outcome. We included dummy variables for age category, application year, and state. For this analysis, data from California included all approvals and denials.

Second, we tabulated counts of denied claims by denial reason if such information was provided. In these analyses, we dropped claims from California that had multiple denial reasons (30.7% of all denied claims from women sexual assault survivors). We fit separate linear probability models to examine racial/ethnic differences in each claim denial for women sexual assault survivors; we coded each denial reason as a binary outcome. Models included dummy variables for age category, application year, and state.

Third, we examined the marginal effect of referral source on eventual claim approvals using data from 4 states that provided referral information: Arizona, Minnesota, Oklahoma, and Texas. This model compared the referral sources in terms of the probability that a woman sexual assault survivor would be compensated, adjusting for race/ethnicity, age, application year, and state. We measured age as a continuous variable, and application years ranged from 2015 through 2022 because of data availability.

We conducted analyses using Stata 18 (StataCorp LP, College Station, TX). All models included robust SEs.

RESULTS

Our analytic sample included 42 902 claims for compensation by women survivors of sexual assault from 18 states, spanning 9 years (2015–2023). Most survivors were aged 18 to 24 years (28.9%) or 25 to 49 years (43.2%); age data were missing for 20.7% of claims. Non-Hispanic White survivors accounted for 42.1% of all claims; 20.8% were from Latina applicants, and 15.1% from non-Hispanic Black applicants (Table 1).

Unadjusted approval rates across racial/ethnic subgroups ranged from 66.5% for Non-Hispanic Indigenous women to 78.5% for Non-Hispanic Asian women. Applications from men were approved less often than those from women: 62.2% versus 74.4%, respectively (Table A). State-level claim approval rates for women ranged from 29.4% in Illinois to 94.1% in New Hampshire (Table B, available as a supplement to the online version of this article at http://www.ajph.org).

In analyses adjusted for age category, state, and application year, claims for Black and Indigenous women were significantly less likely than were those for White women to be approved ($P<.001$; Figure 1). Compensation claims for women aged 25 to 49 or 50 to 64 years were less likely to be approved than were those for women aged 18 to 24 years ($P<.001$). After considering controls, we found that non-Hispanic White women had a 79.9% (95% confidence interval [CI] = 79.2%, 80.5%) probability of approval, whereas non-Hispanic Black and non-Hispanic Indigenous women had 76.5% (95% CI = 75.4%, 77.7%) and 71.9% (95% CI = 68%, 75.9%), respectively, probabilities of approval. The model correctly predicted the approval outcome for 76.9% of claims.[12]

The most common reason for victim compensation claim denial was that law enforcement did not have sufficient evidence to determine that a crime had occurred (34.4% of denials; Figure 2). Other common reasons for claim denial were incomplete applications (25.4%), failure to establish economic loss (8.6%), and failure to cooperate with police (7.8%). Racial/ethnic variation in approval probability appeared to be driven largely by denials for incomplete applications and failure to establish economic loss (Table D, available as a supplement to the online version of this article at http://www.ajph.org).

In analyses of pooled claims from the 4 states that provided data on referral source (Arizona, Minnesota, Oklahoma, and Texas), the predicted probability of approval for claimants referred from hospitals or law enforcement agencies was 66.8% and 68.9%, respectively (Figure 3). Only claimants referred by nonprofit service providers and public advertisements had a

TABLE 1— Characteristics of Women Filing State Victim Compensation Program Claims After Sexual Assault: 18 US States, 2015–2023

Characteristic	Total Claims, No. (%)	Approval Rate, %
Total	42 902 (100)	74.4
Race/ethnicity		
Non-Hispanic White	18 078 (42.1)	75.9
Non-Hispanic Black	6 462 (15.1)	72.2
Latina	8 909 (20.8)	77.0
Non-Hispanic Asian	1 243 (2.9)	78.5
Non-Hispanic Indigenous	556 (1.3)	66.5
Other	1 675 (3.9)	75.8
Missing race/ethnicity	5 979 (13.9)	67.6
Age, y		
18–24	12 406 (28.9)	78.6
25–49	18 532 (43.2)	76.2
50–64	2 629 (6.1)	75.1
≥ 65	471 (1.1)	75.8
Missing age	8 864 (20.7)	64.2

Note. The states included were AZ, CA, FL, GA, IA, IL, MA, MD, MN, ND, NH, NY, OK, RI, TX, WA, WV, and WY. Numbers include cases with claim decisions. Age data were missing for Massachusetts and New York. All claims from Massachusetts were included in the total and race/ethnicity figures. Claims from New York were limited to adults aged 20 years and older, and were included in the total and race/ethnicity figures.

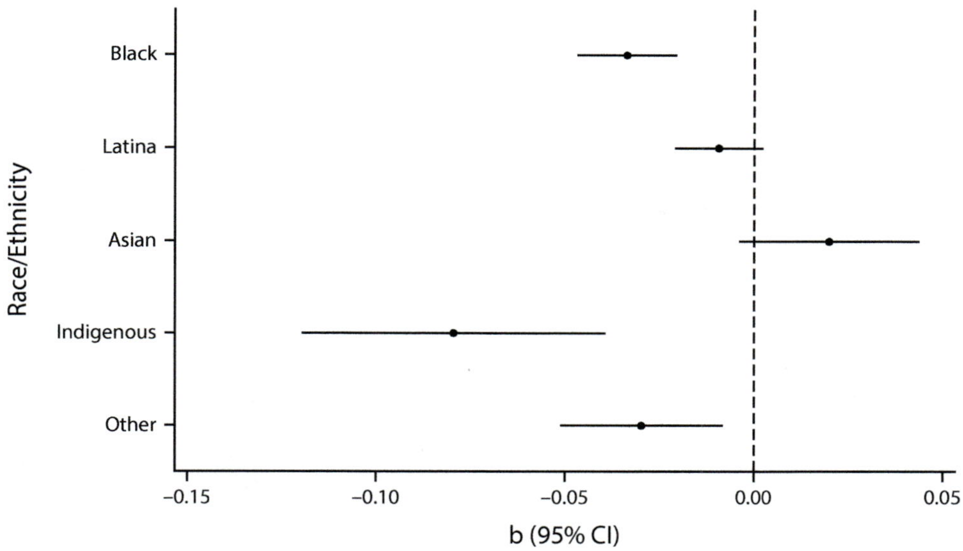

FIGURE 1— Likelihood of Survivor Compensation Claim Approval Among Women by Race/Ethnicity, Adjusted for Age, State, and Application Year: 16 US States, 2015–2023

Note. CI = confidence interval. The states included were AZ, CA, FL, GA, IA, IL, MD, MN, ND, NH, OK, RI, TX, WA, WV, and WY. We excluded claims from MA and NY because of missing or incompatible subgroup categories. Parameter estimates and 95% CIs were derived from a linear probability model regressing sexual assault claim approval on race/ethnicity. (See also Table C, available as a supplement to the online version of this article at http://www.ajph.org.) The reference group was White women.

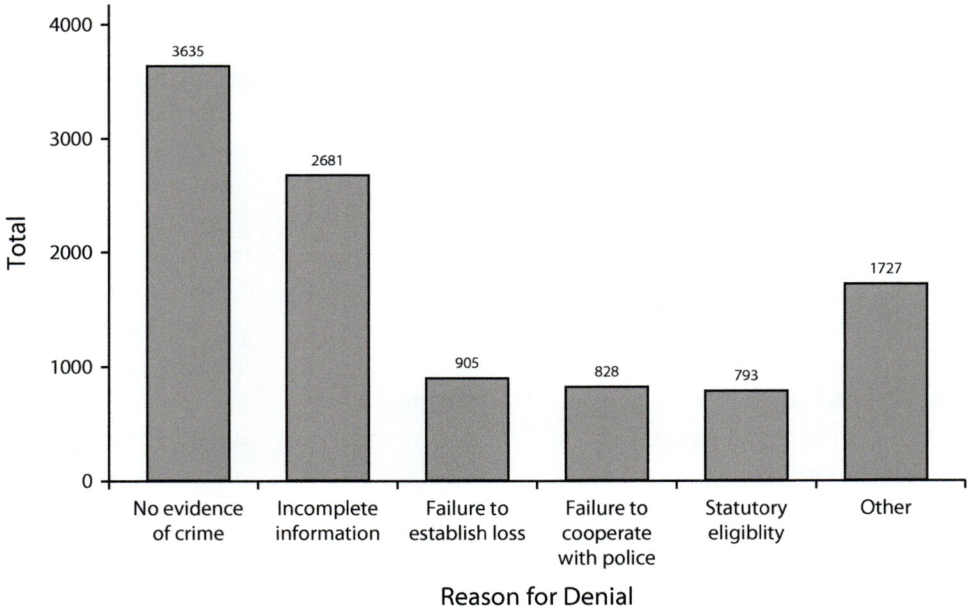

FIGURE 2— Denied Claims for Women Sexual Assault Survivors by Denial Reason: 18 US States, 2015–2023

Note. The states included were AZ, CA, FL, GA, IA, IL, MA, MD, MN, ND, NH, NY, OK, RI, TX, WA, WV, and WY.

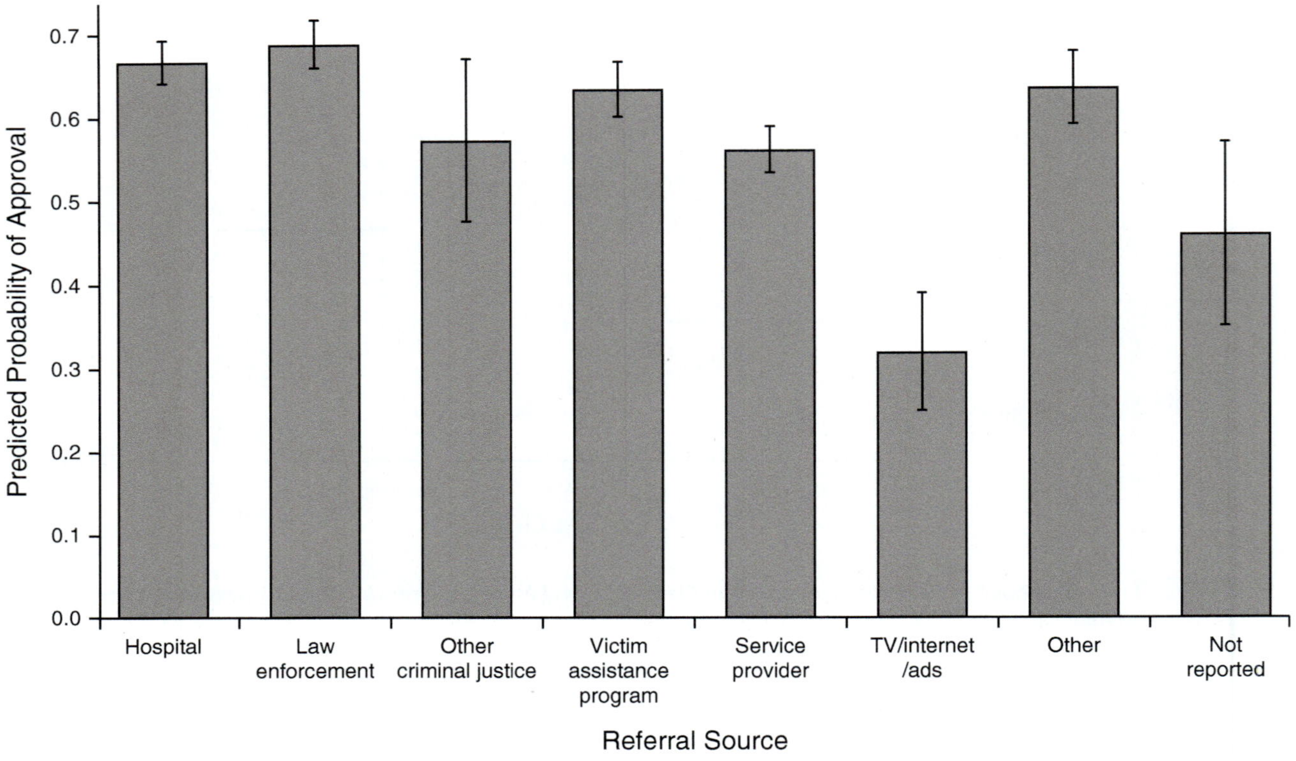

FIGURE 3— Association of Referral Source with Probability of Claim Approval for Women Sexual Assault Survivors: Arizona, Minnesota, Oklahoma, and Texas, 2015–2022

Note. Referral source and claim approval data were available only for AZ, MN, OK, and TX. Bars indicate predicted probabilities. The 95% confidence intervals are shown.

significantly lower probability of approval than claimants referred by hospitals ($P < .001$).

DISCUSSION

Claims by survivors of sexual assault to state victim compensation programs submitted by non-Hispanic Black and non-Hispanic Indigenous women were less likely to be approved than were claims made by non-Hispanic White and non-Hispanic Asian women, even after adjusting for age, application year, and state fixed effects. Racial disparities in approval rates appear to have been driven largely by incomplete applications and other paperwork burdens, underscoring the interplay between race/ethnicity and institutional practices in shaping victim compensation outcomes—an important but understudied safety net for survivors of sexual assault.

The most common reason for claim denials was that the compensation program, informed by law enforcement reports, determined that there was no evidence of a crime. Although there are no estimates of false reporting among people who apply for compensation, overall false reporting of sexual assault is low, with estimates ranging from 4.5% to 5.9%,[13–15] and this is lower than the rate of "no evidence of a crime" denials in our study (8.56%). It is therefore possible that at least some of these determinations are related to outdated assumptions in the criminal legal system about "real rape,"[16] the notion that rape must involve the threat of immediate violent force and be perpetrated by a stranger, rather than by a family member, intimate partner, or someone else known to the survivor.

The prevalence of denials owing to incomplete applications and failure to cooperate with law enforcement highlights the bureaucratic hurdles survivors encounter when seeking compensation. These findings echo previous research on the challenging, sometimes retraumatizing experiences sexual assault survivors face in navigating the criminal legal system.[17] Such disparities align with the concept of racialized organizations, which posits that organizational structures and processes can perpetuate racial inequalities even in the absence of individual bias,[18] especially when decision-making authority is distributed to local jurisdictions.[7]

Language barriers may lead to more claim denials because of incomplete applications, which were more common among Latina women (although we lacked data on claimants' language proficiency, and 15 of 18 states in our study have application forms available in Spanish).

Higher claim approval rates for survivors referred by hospitals and law enforcement, compared with those from other service providers, potentially suggest that victim compensation programs prefer more institutionalized pathways of seeking assistance after sexual assault. This disparity may disadvantage women of color, who—because of long-standing discrimination by both law enforcement[19] and medical institutions[20]—may choose alternative support systems or be hesitant to engage with formal institutions immediately after their assault. Bolstering postemergency visit outreach and direct assistance programs for survivors of trauma may improve access to victim compensation and decrease disparities based on age, housing status, and educational attainment.[21]

The striking state-level variation in claim approval rates was beyond the scope of our study and warrants further analysis. Lower approval rates may be caused by stricter definitions of sexual assault in the criminal legal system or more confusing application paperwork requirements in some states. Policing processes may also affect approval rates. Although approval for compensation does not depend on successful convictions, claims by survivors who recant their criminal complaint (which is common among survivors of domestic violence)[22] or are perceived as uncooperative are more likely to be denied. Survivor cooperation rates may vary by police jurisdiction.

It is additionally possible that states with lower approval rates may support survivors of sexual assault through other sources; states where survivors are more likely to be covered by Medicaid (e.g., Illinois) could have lower approval rates because survivors who would have otherwise been approved for victim compensation may receive medical coverage with minimal out-of-pocket costs through Medicaid instead. Yet we found lower claim approval rates among states with a range of Medicaid policy environments (e.g., Texas, which has not expanded Medicaid, and Maryland, which has). Future research should investigate these and other factors because they may contribute to the uneven implementation of victim compensation across the country.

Recent policy changes in several states offer directions for reform. Illinois passed a law in 2021 that considers hospital visits as satisfying the "cooperation" requirement. Similarly, New York's Fair Access to Victim Compensation Act, signed in 2023, and Maryland's Victim Compensation Reform Act of 2024 both removed police reports from the claims process, mitigating the deterrent effect of mandatory police reporting. Additional reforms aimed at simplifying and standardizing claim applications may decrease administrative barriers and racial disparities in claims made and ultimately approved. In 2024, potential changes to federal guidelines were introduced that would have decreased cooperation requirements, but these proposed changes were withdrawn in January 2025 in anticipation of resistance by the Trump administration.

Our study has limitations, including that we lacked data for states that ignored or denied freedom of information requests. Although most compensation funding at the national level[5] is used for health care services (including forensic medical examinations), we lacked data on allocations at the survivor and claim levels. We also lacked data on survivors' health insurance status. Because victim compensation is a payer of last resort, claimants included both uninsured survivors and insured survivors with out-of-pocket costs because of deductibles and other cost sharing. We also limited our analyses to adult sexual assault survivors because of data availability. Some states classify cases of sexual assault of those younger than 18 years as "child sexual abuse" rather than "sexual assault." Also, the data do not contain enough detail to distinguish claims covering child survivors' medical costs, claims for mental health care for parents of abused children, and claims made by adults who were abused as children. This is another important area for future research.

Additionally, application rates for compensation may differ by racial/ethnic group, and it is possible that White survivors who might have otherwise been denied do not apply, inflating approval rates, although selection effects are more likely to bias our results in the other direction (masking even greater racial disparities), given substantially higher trust in law enforcement (which is likely associated with crime reporting and filing compensation claims) among White versus Black Americans.[23] Finally, resources at the federal level to improve data management systems and data availability would facilitate better public understanding of victim compensation programs and help improve access to support services for survivors of sexual assault and other violent crimes.

Our data do not include claims made by survivors who were sexually assaulted while incarcerated. Most states' compensation programs exclude incarcerated individuals, despite rates of sexual assault that are more than 10 times greater for women in prison than those in the nonincarcerated population.[24]

Victim compensation programs play a crucial role in supporting survivors of sexual assault, yet significant barriers and disparities persist. Addressing these challenges requires both policy reform and institutional change, including a commitment to equitable access despite variation in survivors' reporting preferences. AJPH

ABOUT THE AUTHORS

Samuel Dickman is with Planned Parenthood of Montana, Billings. Jeremy Levine is with the Departments of Organizational Studies and Sociology, University of Michigan, Ann Arbor. Chalem Bolton was with the Department of Sociology, University of Michigan, Ann Arbor, at the time of this study. Anna Conway is with the Department of Organizational Studies, University of Michigan. Kelly Russell is with the Department of Sociology, Florida State University, Tallahassee.

CORRESPONDENCE

Correspondence should be sent to Samuel Dickman, MD, 1844 Broadwater Ave #4, Billings, MT 59102 (e-mail: samuel.dickman@ppmontana.org). Reprints can be ordered at https://www.ajph.org by clicking the "Reprints" link.

PUBLICATION INFORMATION

Full Citation: Dickman S, Levine J, Bolton C, Conway A, Russell K. Racial disparities in victim compensation program claim approvals for adult survivors of sexual assault: 18 US states, 2015–2023. *Am J Public Health*. 2026;116(3): 380–386.

Acceptance Date: September 25, 2025.

DOI: https://doi.org/10.2105/AJPH.2025.308304

ORCID iDs:

Samuel Dickman https://orcid.org/0000-0003-3126-786X

Chalem Bolton https://orcid.org/0000-0003-0240-2778

CONTRIBUTORS

S. Dickman and J. Levine contributed equally to the article; they designed the study, conducted the analyses, and drafted the article. J. Levine acquired the data. All authors interpreted the data, revised the article critically for intellectual content, and approved the version to be published.

CONFLICTS OF INTEREST

The authors have no conflicts of interest to disclose.

HUMAN PARTICIPANT PROTECTION

This study was not considered human participants research because the data were not collected specifically for the study and no member of the research team had access to participant identifiers.

REFERENCES

1. Leemis RW, Friar N, Khatiwada S, et al. The National Intimate Partner and Sexual Violence Survey: 2016/2017 report on intimate partner violence. October 2022. Available at: https://www.cdc.gov/violenceprevention/pdf/2016-2017-nisvs-report.pdf. Accessed November 26, 2025.
2. Dickman SL, Himmelstein G, Himmelstein DU, et al. Uncovered medical bills after sexual assault. *N Engl J Med*. 2022;387(11):1043–1044. https://doi.org/10.1056/NEJMc2207644
3. Tennessee AM, Bradham TS, White BM, Simpson KN. The monetary cost of sexual assault to privately insured US women in 2013. *Am J Public Health*. 2017;107(6):983–988. https://doi.org/10.2105/AJPH.2017.303742
4. Tapp SN, Coen EJ. Criminal victimization, 2023. September 1, 2024. Available at: https://www.ojp.gov/library/publications/criminal-victimization-2023. Accessed November 26, 2025.
5. Office for Victims of Crime. Victims of Crime Act victim compensation formula grant program. 2020. Available at: https://ovc.ojp.gov/sites/g/files/xyckuh226/files/media/document/fy-2019-voca-compensation-performance-report.pdf. Accessed November 26, 2025.
6. Levine JR. Whose victimization pays? Policing innocent victimhood in victim compensation law. *Law Soc Rev*. 2025:1–37. https://doi.org/10.1017/lsr.2025.10046
7. Planty M, Langton L, Krebs C, Berzofsky M, Smiley-McDonald H. Female victims of sexual violence, 1994–2010. March 2013. Available at: https://bjs.ojp.gov/content/pub/pdf/fvsv9410.pdf. Accessed November 26, 2025.
8. Fording RC, Soss J, Schram SF. Race and the local politics of punishment in the new world of welfare. *AJS*. 2011;116(5):1610–1657. https://doi.org/10.1086/657525
9. Moos EF, Kvasnovsky C, Nordgren R, et al. Twice harmed: a descriptive analysis of Illinois crime victim compensation after sexual assault and domestic violence. *J Surg Res*. 2025;308:279–285. https://doi.org/10.1016/j.jss.2025.02.036
10. Adcock C. Uncompensated loss: Black families of murder victims more likely to be denied aid from state program. *The Frontier*. July 9, 2019. Available at: https://www.readfrontier.org/stories/uncompensated-loss-black-homicide-victims-more-likely-to-be-denied-funds-from-a-state-program-to-help-victims-of-violent-crime-data-shows. Accessed November 26, 2025.
11. Lumley T, Diehr P, Emerson S, Chen L. The importance of the normality assumption in large public health data sets. *Annu Rev Public Health*. 2002;23:151–169. https://doi.org/10.1146/annurev.publhealth.23.100901.140546
12. Wooldridge JM. *Introductory Econometrics: A Modern Approach*. Boston, MA: Cengage Learning; 2016.
13. Lisak D, Gardinier L, Nicksa SC, Cote AM. False allegations of sexual assault: an analysis of ten years of reported cases. *Violence Against Women*. 2010;16(12):1318–1334. https://doi.org/10.1177/1077801210387747
14. Ferguson CE, Malouff JM. Assessing police classifications of sexual assault reports: a meta-analysis of false reporting rates. *Arch Sex Behav*. 2016;45(5):1185–1193. https://doi.org/10.1007/s10508-015-0666-2
15. Spohn C, White C, Tellis K. Unfounding sexual assault: examining the decision to unfound and identifying false reports. *Law Soc Rev*. 2014;48(1): 161–192. https://doi.org/10.1111/lasr.12060
16. Estrich S. *Real Rape*. Cambridge, MA: Harvard University Press; 1987.
17. Campbell R. The psychological impact of rape victims. *Am Psychol*. 2008;63(8):702–717. https://doi.org/10.1037/0003-066X.63.8.702
18. Ray V. A theory of racialized organizations. *Am Sociol Rev*. 2019;84(1):26–53. https://doi.org/10.1177/0003122418822335
19. Bor J, Venkataramani AS, Williams DR, Tsai AC. Police killings and their spillover effects on the mental health of Black Americans: a population-based, quasi-experimental study. *Lancet*. 2018; 392(10144):302–310. https://doi.org/10.1016/S0140-6736(18)31130-9
20. Chandran M, Schulman KA. Racial disparities in healthcare and health. *Health Serv Res*. 2022; 57(2):218–222. https://doi.org/10.1111/1475-6773.13957
21. Alvidrez J, Shumway M, Boccellari A, Green JD, Kelly V, Merrill G. Reduction of state victim compensation disparities in disadvantaged crime victims through active outreach and assistance: a randomized trial. *Am J Public Health*. 2008;98(5): 882–888. https://doi.org/10.2105/AJPH.2007.113639
22. Bonomi AE, Gangamma R, Locke CR, Katafiasz H, Martin D. "Meet me at the hill where we used to park": interpersonal processes associated with victim recantation. *Soc Sci Med*. 2011;73(7): 1054–1061. https://doi.org/10.1016/j.socscimed.2011.07.005
23. Morin R, Stepler R. The racial confidence gap in police performance. September 29, 2016. Available at: https://www.pewresearch.org/social-trends/2016/09/29/the-racial-confidence-gap-in-police-performance. Accessed November 26, 2025.
24. Wolff N, Blitz CL, Shi J, Bachman R, Siegel JA. Sexual violence inside prisons: rates of victimization. *J Urban Health*. 2006;83(5):835–848. https://doi.org/10.1007/s11524-006-9065-2

Bridging the Hearing Divide: Policy Solutions for Aging Americans

Meghana Rajashekara Swamy, MD, MPH, MS, Richard Marottoli, MD, MPH, and Andrew B. Cohen, MD, DPhil

Hearing loss affects approximately two thirds of adults in the United States aged 70 years or older and frequently remains untreated despite its well-documented harms, including accelerated cognitive decline, increased caregiver burden, and higher health care expenditures.

We examine the major barriers to accessing high-quality hearing care, with particular attention to the complex and fragmented landscape of insurance coverage across Medicare, Medicaid, the US Department of Veterans Affairs, private plans, and over-the-counter (OTC) products. We review key legislative and regulatory developments over the past decade, most notably the 2022 establishment of OTC hearing aids, and summarize early opportunities and remaining gaps. We then propose targeted reforms to improve access and affordability, including more consistent Medicaid benefits, selective Medicare expansion, integration of teleaudiology, and strengthened oversight and consumer protections for OTC devices. Finally, we advance a technology-driven policy framework that integrates artificial intelligence–supported risk prediction, teleaudiology, real-time insurance verification, and a transparent device marketplace to modernize delivery and evaluation.

Together, these strategies can catalyze a fundamental rethinking of how hearing health is prioritized and managed within the broader United States health care ecosystem. (*Am J Public Health*. 2026;116(3): 387–396. https://doi.org/10.2105/AJPH.2025.308298)

AJPH March 2026, Vol. 116, No. 3

Nearly two thirds of adults aged 70 years or older in the United States experience hearing loss, with the prevalence rising sharply from 45% among those 70 to 74 years of age to more than 80% among those aged 85 years and older.[1,2] Hearing loss is associated with cognitive decline, social isolation, diminished quality of life, safety concerns, and poorer mental health outcomes.[2–5] Despite its prevalence and well-documented consequences, access to effective hearing health care, including hearing aids, remains constrained by gaps in health insurance coverage and systemic policy barriers.[2]

The 2016 National Academies of Sciences, Engineering, and Medicine (NASEM) report *Hearing Health Care for Adults: Priorities for Improving Access and Affordability* identified critical barriers to hearing health care, including the high cost of hearing aids, inadequate insurance coverage, and limited public awareness of hearing loss.[2] The report recommended enhancing access, affordability, and integration of hearing care within public health.[2] Since the publication of the NASEM report, legislative changes, the advent of over-the-counter (OTC) hearing aids, and growing evidence of the cognitive and social benefits of early intervention collectively underscore the need to update policy recommendations to address persistent disparities in hearing health care access.[3,5,6]

This article offers 3 key contributions for policymakers, researchers, and public health stakeholders. First, it updates the policy landscape since the 2016 NASEM report, highlighting the Food and Drug Administration (FDA) 2022 rule permitting OTC hearing aids for mild to moderate hearing loss and recent actions by the Centers for Medicare & Medicaid Services (CMS) to expand audiology access for Medicare beneficiaries.

Second, it examines persistent gaps in insurance coverage, including Medicare's exclusion of hearing aids, the limited uptake of Medicare Advantage benefits, state-level variability in Medicaid coverage, geographic restrictions in Veterans Affairs (VA) benefits, and the inconsistent and costly nature of private insurance. It also reviews financing strategies such as standardized benefit criteria, payer–government risk sharing, and bundled payments.

Third, it proposes a framework for improving access to hearing care through digital technologies and artificial intelligence across the continuum of service delivery. This framework emphasizes practical tools such as risk prediction, mobile self-assessment, telehealth rehabilitation, and real-time insurance navigation, all supported by safeguards for privacy, equity, and interoperability.

AGING AND UNTREATED HEARING LOSS: PUBLIC HEALTH IMPLICATIONS

In the United States, the population aged 65 years and older is expected to reach 82 million by 2050, a 47% increase from 50 million in 2022.[7] This demographic surge amplifies concerns about untreated hearing loss, which is linked to higher risks of cognitive decline and dementia.[8,9] In turn, these health effects intensify public health challenges by escalating health care costs, increasing program expenditures for aging services, and elevating caregiver burden.[10] Given the global increase in dementia cases to approximately 153 million in 2025, with hearing loss contributing to 7% of these cases, the need for targeted audiological interventions to mitigate cognitive decline has become increasingly relevant.[8,9]

Beyond dementia, untreated hearing loss may increase safety risks; although evidence is mixed, some studies link it to higher rates of falls and motor vehicle crashes, likely through impaired perception of environmental cues.[4,11] Moreover, communication difficulties exacerbate caregiver burden and stress, creating an often-overlooked strain on familial and informal care networks.[12] Audiological care, including access to hearing aids, can help contain these individual and caregiver health-related costs by preserving functional independence.[2,4,12]

Economically, untreated hearing loss hinders individuals' employment prospects and job retention, leading to greater financial instability.[13] This dynamic not only diminishes quality of life but also strains health care systems through a higher reliance on social welfare programs.[2,10,13] Conversely, improving hearing aid accessibility enhances self-sufficiency and workplace productivity, thereby contributing to economic stability for both aging populations and health care infrastructures.[2,13]

The Aging and Cognitive Health Evaluation in Elders (ACHIEVE) trial, a landmark multicenter randomized controlled study, offers particularly compelling evidence regarding the benefits of early hearing intervention.[9] ACHIEVE enrolled older adults with mild to moderate hearing loss from 2 cohorts, participants from the Atherosclerosis Risk in Communities study and a newly recruited community sample.[9] Participants were randomly assigned to receive either immediate hearing care, including hearing aids fitted by audiologists, or a successful aging intervention as the control condition.[9] During 3 years of follow-up, participants from the Atherosclerosis Risk in Communities cohort (at elevated risk for cognitive decline) who received timely hearing aids had a 48% lower risk of cognitive decline than those not involved in the intervention.[9] By combining standardized audiological and neurocognitive measures, ACHIEVE demonstrated that hearing interventions preserve cognition and are cost-effective in reducing dementia risk.[9]

Data from the 2003–2004 National Health and Nutrition Examination Survey demonstrate a clear gradient in hearing loss by income and education: adults in the lowest income quartile had 1.64 times the odds of bilateral hearing impairment (95% confidence interval [CI] = 1.09, 2.47) compared with those in the highest quartile, and individuals without a high school diploma had significantly greater odds of high-frequency hearing loss than college graduates.[14] These findings highlight resource-driven disparities in audiological care and risk factor exposure.[14] Therefore, addressing hearing health is a public health imperative closely linked to health equity and resource optimization.[2,14]

ASSESSING RECENT DEVELOPMENTS IN EVIDENCE AND POLICY

This analytic essay synthesizes recent developments in US hearing health policy. In doing so, we initially conducted an unstructured review of peer-reviewed publications, policy analyses, and legislative and regulatory documents published between July 2008 and May 2025. To ensure a comprehensive view of the current policy environment, we also consulted Web sites and resources from key agencies and organizations including the FDA, the CMS, the Centers for Disease Control and Prevention, NASEM, state Medicaid agencies, and the Kaiser Family Foundation.

The evidence was organized into 4 broad domains (policy, device type, service modality, and cross-cutting themes) and examined in terms of relevance to access, coverage, financing, and equity. The findings were triangulated across the peer-reviewed literature, regulatory documents, policy analyses, and Web sites, with cross checking across independent sources to strengthen reliability and consistency. The search strategy, including databases used, key terms, and inclusion criteria, is described in more detail in the Appendix (available as a supplement to the online version of this article at http://www.ajph.org). A list of key sources by domain is provided in Appendix Table A, which serves as a compact evidence map of the literature informing US hearing health policy. The complete set of 37 sources, classified by publication type, subtype, and year of publication, is presented in Appendix Table B. The temporal distribution of these sources is shown in Appendix Figure A.

REVIEW OF EVIDENCE

Systemic barriers continue to restrict older adults' access to high-quality audiologic care, thereby limiting hearing aid use.[2,15] As of 2019, fewer than one third of adults aged 70 years and older who could benefit from hearing aids had ever used them.[2,16,17] The 2021 National Health Interview Survey revealed a similarly low usage rate of 14.4% among adults aged 65 years and older, with men more likely than women to use hearing aids.[18]

Hearing Health Access in the United States

Low rates of use of hearing aids stem from multiple interdependent factors. Restricted access to audiological care, primarily driven by high costs and variable insurance coverage, remains a key barrier.[2,19] Limited awareness of hearing care needs, low self-perceived need for hearing aid use, and uncertainty about coverage options further discourage individuals from seeking treatment.[18–20] Even among those who obtain hearing aids, insufficient patient education, training, and follow-up by health care professionals can compromise device effectiveness.[2,19,20] Solutions to these issues include individualized device fitting, patient education and training, and clear information on coverage and services.[2]

The introduction of OTC hearing aids, following the FDA's final rule published in August 2022 and implemented in October 2022, has markedly enhanced affordability and accessibility for adults with perceived mild to moderate hearing loss.[6,21] This regulatory change enables consumers to purchase hearing aids directly without requiring a prescription or an initial professional evaluation, thereby reducing cost barriers and expediting access.[6,21] Furthermore, updated coverage guidelines from the CMS, as outlined in the 2023 Physician Fee Schedule Final Rule, have streamlined audiology service referral processes, further expanding access to hearing care.[22] Box 1 provides an overview of recent advancements in hearing health care access.

However, despite these advancements, notable limitations persist. OTC devices typically exclude professional services such as fitting, calibration, and audiological rehabilitation, rendering them unsuitable for individuals with severe hearing loss (who represent 4.2% of adults aged 71 years and older according to the 2021 National Health Aging and Trends Study) and potentially exacerbating disparities in care.[6,17,21] Moreover, many older adults, particularly those with multiple comorbidities, require comprehensive audiological evaluations to optimize device programming and ensure long-term adherence.[2,6,17,21]

BOX 1— Recent Developments in Hearing Health Care Access

Development	Year(s)	Key Provisions	Potential Impact
FDA authorization of OTC hearing aids	2022	• Final rule published in August 2022 and implemented in October 2022.[6,21] • Permits direct, prescription-free purchase of hearing aids for mild to moderate loss.[6,21] • Eliminates the need for an initial professional evaluation.[6,21]	• Reduces cost barriers and expedites access to hearing care.[6,21,34] • Supports early intervention but may be less suitable for severe or complex hearing loss.[6,21]
CMS revised guidelines and referral protocols	2022–2023	• Updates outlined in the 2023 Physician Fee Schedule Final Rule streamline audiology service referral processes.[22] • Expands access to hearing care for Medicare beneficiaries by reducing the administrative barrier of obtaining a physician referral.[22]	• Medicare beneficiaries can directly access 36 specific audiology services for nonacute hearing conditions without a physician or nonphysician practitioner order once every 12 months.[22]

Note. CMS = Centers for Medicare & Medicaid Services; FDA = Food and Drug Administration; OTC = over the counter.

In addition, although the revised CMS guidelines and streamlined referral protocols have improved access, challenges persist as they apply only to a restricted set of 36 Current Procedural Terminology codes for nonacute, gradually progressive hearing loss and exclude coverage for hearing aid assessment, fitting, acquisition, and ongoing care.[22] All other audiology services, including the aforementioned, continue to require an order from a physician or nonphysician practitioner.[22] This inconsistency frequently leads to out-of-pocket costs for patients and creates administrative burdens for providers, particularly in settings with limited audiology support.[20,22] Thus, simply supplying a hearing aid, whether OTC or not, cannot surmount these barriers; a comprehensive hearing care model that includes professional assessments, precise device fitting, rehabilitative services, and ongoing follow-up is essential to fully leverage the benefits of amplification.[2]

These utilization challenges underscore the limitations of current service models and highlight the need for policy updates that address inconsistencies in coverage and ensure ongoing support for hearing aid users.[2,19] The sections to follow examine how insurance frameworks and regulatory practices contribute to these barriers and offer actionable strategies to improve hearing care access and affordability.

Insurance and OTC Hearing Aids: Gaps and Advances

Medicaid coverage for hearing aids varies substantially across states, creating geographic disparities in access unrelated to medical need and preventing many low-income older adults from accessing hearing care.[2] Although the Affordable Care Act expanded Medicaid in many states and mandates coverage for essential health benefits, it does not require hearing aid coverage, leaving this benefit optional.[2,23,24] For example, California's Medi-Cal covers hearing aids for adults aged 65 years and older and requires an audiological evaluation and physician prescription.[25] Coverage includes a $1510 annual cap and prior authorization for expenses exceeding $254.[25] By contrast, neighboring Arizona's Medicaid program offers no coverage for hearing aids for older adults.[26] The Build Back Better Act, proposed in 2021, included reforms to expand hearing aid coverage that would have substantially improved access for Medicaid beneficiaries; however, although it passed the House of Representatives, it failed to advance in the Senate and ultimately did not become law.[27]

Medicare's lack of hearing aid coverage results in high out-of-pocket costs for older adults that limit access to essential audiological care.[2,17] Traditional Medicare excludes coverage for hearing aids and routine hearing examinations, requiring beneficiaries to cover these costs entirely.[2,17,28] This coverage gap has persisted for decades without substantive policy intervention.[17,28]

Medicare Part B does cover diagnostic hearing exams when ordered by a physician to determine the need for medical treatment.[2,28] According to the policy introduced in January 2023 by the CMS, patients can directly access audiologists for diagnostic tests related to nonacute hearing conditions once every 12 months without requiring a physician's referral.[2,22] Despite this change, the policy continues to exclude services related to hearing aids and examinations for prescribing, fitting, or adjusting hearing aids.[2,22] Consequently, beneficiaries must seek coverage through Medicare Advantage plans or pay out of pocket.[2,17,20,29]

Although 97% of Medicare Advantage plans offer hearing benefits, utilization remains low, with only 5% of enrollees undergoing routine hearing tests, 4% receiving hearing aid fittings, and just over 2% purchasing hearing aids.[17,18,29] Several factors may contribute to this low uptake. Many beneficiaries are unaware of their coverage.[20] In addition, out-of-pocket costs, including copays and limited allowances for hearing aids, deter use.[2,20,29] Complex plan structures, such as restrictions on covered providers and variability in benefit design, pose further barriers.[2,20]

Two recent legislative proposals aimed at improving Medicare hearing aid coverage for older adults failed to be passed into law. The Medicare Hearing Aid Coverage Act, introduced in the House in February 2021 to expand Medicare benefits for hearing aids, did not progress beyond the committee stage.[30] The Build Back Better Act also contained provisions to expand Medicare coverage for hearing care services; however, these measures were not enacted as the bill stalled in the Senate.[27]

The VA hearing aid program provides free devices and services to eligible veterans, but challenges remain in ensuring timely and convenient access to these services.[31] Geographic barriers, particularly for rural veterans who often live far from specialized hearing care facilities, are a major issue.[31] Although VA coverage has increased hearing aid usage and remote care initiatives have begun to alleviate these challenges, additional improvements are necessary to enhance access to hearing care.[31] Potential measures include the distribution of low-cost devices for all veterans, expanded broadband access in rural areas, and the development of integrated smartphone applications with user-friendly interfaces for remote hearing assessments.[32]

Private health insurance provides limited coverage for hearing aids, typically as optional add-ons.[23] High out-of-pocket costs, with an average bundled price of $2500, make hearing aids financially inaccessible for 77% of Americans with hearing loss; among those who would need to pay such an amount, an estimated 4% could be pushed into poverty.[2,23,33]

The FDA's approval of OTC hearing aids represents a pivotal step in addressing accessibility gaps by eliminating the need for prescriptions or audiologist fittings.[6] Although OTC devices have expanded access for many, their overall effectiveness remains under evaluation; cost-effectiveness analyses suggest that OTC hearing aids must deliver at least 55% of the utility benefit of traditional devices to be considered a viable alternative.[34] Moreover, because OTC devices are unsuitable for severe hearing loss, they leave a coverage gap for those with the greatest need.[6,33,34] In addition, recent assessments have raised important consumer protection concerns.[2,35] Issues such as misleading product labeling, questionable FDA certifications, and the lack of robust mechanisms for recourse in cases of defective or ineffective devices underscore the need for enhanced regulatory oversight.[2,35] Comprehensive policy reforms to close regulatory gaps and strengthen consumer safeguards are essential for equitable, effective hearing care.[2,35,36]

Box 2 offers a comparative analysis of hearing aid coverage, patterns of use, access disparities, out-of-pocket costs, and population reach across different insurance models and OTC devices. The data show marked disparities in coverage, costs, and utilization, underscoring systemic inequities. Note that this wide variation in costs results from differences in insurance coverage, such as state-specific Medicaid benefit caps or the complete absence of hearing aid benefits in some states.[23,25,26] Traditional Medicare excludes routine hearing aid coverage, leaving older adults to cover full costs, whereas private insurance varies in benefit design and OTC devices are sold at unregulated prices.[2,23,28,29,34]

ANALYSIS

A multifaceted approach that addresses policy gaps, insurance limitations, and care delivery challenges is important for enhancing hearing health access among older adults in the United States. This will require strategies to optimize coverage, affordability, and service integration.[2,13]

Implementation Barriers: Analysis and Strategy

Federal Medicaid mandates with targeted reimbursement incentives could help make hearing aid coverage more consistent across states and reduce geographic disparities; however, budget constraints and administrative complexities remain challenges.[2,23] A potential solution is a federal and state cost-sharing model that improves the existing Federal Medical Assistance Percentage formula specifically for hearing services.[37] For instance, implementing an initial 90% federal match for hearing services alongside federally established baseline coverage standards could promote greater consistency.[37] Although an enhanced federal and state cost-sharing model may initially seem costly, this model would incorporate cost-containment measures by linking additional funding to measurable performance outcomes, thereby incentivizing states to adopt efficient, cost-effective practices.[2,37] Targeted grant funding for community education and outreach would further ensure that expenditures directly enhance access to hearing care.[2,20] Over time, improved health outcomes may yield long-term health care savings that offset initial investments.[2,13]

Expanding traditional Medicare coverage to include routine hearing exams and hearing aids, coupled with sliding-scale subsidies that adjust support according to individual income and need, could greatly improve affordability.[2,24,28] Although current federal budget constraints may make full coverage impractical, targeted subsidies could ensure that lower-income beneficiaries receive necessary assistance.[2,14,16] To address challenges such as provider shortages and long wait times, one strategy might be to incentivize the expansion of the audiology workforce through scholarships, loan forgiveness programs, and residency expansion for audiology training.[2,28,29] Improving timely, high-quality hearing care can prevent falls, cognitive decline, and hospitalizations, lowering long-term costs and improving outcomes.[2–4]

Particularly for rural and mobility-limited older adults, integrating tele-audiology services into Medicare and Medicaid, building on the VA model, could improve access and reduce costs.[31,32] However, infrastructure deficiencies and digital literacy barriers among older adults may limit adoption.[32] Expanding broadband access and investing in targeted digital training

AJPH March 2026, Vol. 116, No. 3

BOX 2— Comparative Analysis of Hearing Aid Coverage, Use, Access, Costs, and Population Reach Across Insurance Models and OTC Devices

Insurance Type	Coverage Details	Use Challenges	Out-of-Pocket Costs	Population Coverage
Medicaid	• Coverage varies by state; some states offer partial or full benefits, whereas others provide no benefits.[2,23,25,26]	• Substantial geographic disparities in coverage because of state-level variations.[2,23] • Prior authorization for expenses and caps on coverage limit accessibility.[2,23]	• Some states impose annual caps (e.g., $1510 in California), and many provide no coverage at all.[25,26]	• Approximately 40%–50% of low-income individuals in states with Medicaid hearing aid benefits.[16–19]
Medicare	• Traditional Medicare does not cover routine hearing exams or hearing aids.[28] • Diagnostic exams are covered under Part B only when ordered by a physician.[28,29] • Medicare Advantage plans may offer hearing benefits, but use remains low.[28,29]	• High out-of-pocket costs persist, with only 5% of Medicare Advantage enrollees undergoing routine hearing tests and just 2% purchasing hearing aids.[16,18,29]	• Hearing aids cost between $2500 and $6000, with 100% of the cost paid by beneficiaries unless covered under Medicare Advantage.[2,29,33]	• Among adults aged 65 years or older, nearly 100% are Medicare beneficiaries.[16–18] • About 50% of Medicare beneficiaries are enrolled in Medicare Advantage plans, but only 14.4% of adults aged 65 years or older report using hearing aids.[16–18]
VA	• Eligible veterans receive free hearing aids and audiology services through the VA.[31,32] • However, rural veterans face access barriers.[31,32]	• Despite free hearing aids, use remains low, especially among rural veterans.[31] • Barriers include uncertainty about access and individuals declining hearing aids because of cost concerns.[31] • Telehealth aims to improve access, but infrastructure challenges persist.[31,32]	• Hearing aids are free for eligible veterans, but travel costs pose financial burdens, especially for rural veterans with limited VA access.[31]	• Approximately 70% of eligible veterans are enrolled in VA health care.[31,32] • Among veterans with self-reported hearing loss, 66.9% have sought hearing care.[31]
Private Insurance	• Coverage is optional with high out-of-pocket costs, and few plans offer comprehensive hearing aid benefits.[2,23,33]	• High out-of-pocket costs deter utilization; only a small percentage of individuals with hearing loss have employer-based or private insurance coverage.[2,23,33]	• $2000–$3500 for basic hearing aid devices; optional plans have high premiums and copays.[2,23,33]	• Only 20% of individuals with hearing loss have private insurance coverage.[2,23,33]
OTC hearing aids	• Designed for mild-to-moderate hearing loss, available without a prescription.[6] • Effectiveness varies, with ongoing regulatory concerns.[6,35]	• Limited consumer safeguards, potential fraud risks, and uncertain efficacy for individuals with severe hearing loss; the issue of a comprehensive hearing care ecosystem remains unaddressed.[6,21,35]	• OTC hearing aids range from $500 to $1200 per device, varying by features and brand.[6,34,35]	• OTC hearing aids could benefit millions with mild to moderate hearing loss, but adoption remains low; only 2% of adults with hearing difficulties have purchased one, and 4% plan to do so within a year.[18,19,21]

Note. OTC = over the counter; VA = Veterans Affairs.

programs could extend the reach of hearing care services and reduce travel-related barriers for older adults in rural areas.[20,32] Timely access to hearing care could reduce the harms of untreated impairment and ease federal health care costs in growing high-risk populations.[2,8,10]

Despite expanded coverage under Medicare Advantage, hearing services remain underused. Targeted outreach efforts, conducted in collaboration with local community health centers and senior advocacy organizations, could improve awareness and help beneficiaries navigate their benefits.[2,20,23,29] Integrating teleaudiology services into Medicare Advantage networks could help reduce travel-related barriers to hearing care for rural populations.[20,22,32] Moreover, Medicare Advantage plans could form public–private partnerships with hearing aid manufacturers, state agencies, and community organizations to offer rebates, bulk purchasing, and subsidized hearing centers, reducing costs and out-of-pocket expenses.[2,29,33]

Effective OTC hearing aid implementation requires monitoring outcomes and ensuring insurance coverage for rehabilitation and fitting to preserve efficacy and affordability.[2,6,34,35] However, associated enforcement costs and persistent concerns, such as misleading product labels and unverified performance claims, have the potential to undermine regulatory oversight and erode consumer confidence.[2,35] To address these challenges, public awareness campaigns should provide clear, evidence-based information through standardized educational materials, webinars, and community workshops while provider-led education programs guide consumers in selecting and using their devices appropriately.[2,36] Implementing robust quality assurance measures, such as independent product testing and clearly defined performance benchmarks, would streamline regulatory oversight by establishing standardized compliance criteria.[2,35,36] Leveraging third-party verification by accredited external organizations would allow regulatory agencies to monitor compliance with safety and performance standards more efficiently, minimizing the need for resource-intensive oversight.[2,35,36]

Motivating private insurance to improve hearing care coverage could involve targeted, incremental changes rather than large-scale reform.[2,23,24] Specifically, providing modest tax incentives to employers that voluntarily expand their employee hearing coverage could promote broader participation without placing substantial burdens on federal budgets.[2,23,33,36] In addition, encouraging insurers to adopt standardized benefit criteria, eligibility thresholds, covered device types, and minimum rehabilitative services would promote consistency across plans.[2,23,33,35] Structured insurer–government risk sharing, tied to outcomes and cost metrics, could sustainably incentivize coverage.[2,33,36]

Targeted pilot programs could be implemented in select regions with unmet hearing care needs to test innovative payment and service delivery models.[2,8,9,20] For example, a bundled payment could cover diagnostics through follow-up (fitting, rehabilitation) with provider–payer risk sharing.[2,33,36] These pilots would collect data on patient outcomes, service use, and cost metrics to compare against traditional fee-for-service models.[2,33,36] These data would guide cost-effectiveness assessments and performance-based reimbursement.[2,33,36] If successful, such a model would provide a scalable blueprint for improving service delivery and reducing economic burdens without imposing additional costs on the federal government.[2,33,36]

Solutions From Emerging Technologies

To address persisting gaps in access, coverage, and affordability, we propose a technology-enabled framework that integrates digital tools, artificial intelligence, and real-time insurance verification across the hearing care continuum for older adults. Machine learning models trained on deidentified or consented electronic health records, pharmacy data, and claims would identify and stratify risk according to clinical, behavioral, and demographic indicators (e.g., ototoxic medications, comorbidities, social isolation, missed visits, audiometric data), recalibrating as new information arrives to target resources efficiently. Predictive analytics would operate under strict privacy safeguards with patient agency over data use, transparent consent, audit trails, and compliance with the Health Insurance Portability and Accountability Act and related regulations.

Scalable, low-cost self-assessment tools, mobile hearing tests, and adaptive questionnaires would be deployed via smartphones, loaned tablets, and secure community kiosks to triage candidates, reduce unnecessary referrals, and reserve audiologists for complex cases. Telehealth visits, asynchronous fitting and rehabilitation, and scheduling algorithms would expand capacity and lower travel and facility costs.

Real-time insurance navigation would query Medicare, Medicaid, and private-payer application programming interfaces to check eligibility, prefill forms, and submit authorizations; blockchain-based smart contracts could automate approvals, cut overhead, accelerate reimbursement, and reduce denials. A government-certified device marketplace would provide price transparency, bulk purchase rebates, standardized reporting, and targeted subsidies for low-income users. To promote digital equity, touchscreen kiosks and digital health coaches in rural and low-income areas would offer multilingual support and accessibility features for users with vision or dexterity challenges. Continuous improvement would rely on anonymized outcome data shared with regulators and payers to flag substandard products, misleading advertising, or inequities. Financial viability would be anchored in public–private alignment, with bundled-payment pilots and performance-based contracts to support risk sharing and value-based care. To maximize effectiveness and impact, the approach should be tested in real-world settings and scaled systematically. Box 3 summarizes the key challenges and proposed strategies related to enhancing health care coverage for hearing health services.

BOX 3— Implementation Challenges and Solutions for Expanding Hearing Health Access

Health Care Coverage Policy Reform	Implementation Challenges	Solutions
Medicaid coverage	• State budget constraints may limit expansion of Medicaid benefits without supplemental federal funding.[2,23] • Administrative challenges include variability in state Medicaid programs and difficulties integrating new mandates into existing frameworks.[2,23,24]	• Adopt a federal–state cost-sharing model that improves the FMAP formula for hearing services, including an initial 90% federal match.[2,37] • Establish baseline coverage standards through federal guidelines.[2,37] • Provide targeted grant-based funding and performance-based incentives to encourage state participation.[2,13,37]
Medicare and Medicare Advantage hearing aid access and coverage	• A limited audiology workforce, insufficient training programs, and high patient demand contribute to longer appointment wait times, particularly in rural and underserved areas.[17,20,28,29] • Low use of hearing services in Medicare Advantage plans persists despite available coverage.[17,29]	• Incentivize expansion of the audiology workforce—through scholarships, loan forgiveness, and residency expansion—to address provider shortages and long wait times.[2,29,36] • For Medicare Advantage beneficiaries, outreach through community health centers and senior advocacy organizations can boost awareness.[2,29,36] • Integrating teleaudiology can reduce travel costs for rural patients.[20,32] • Public–private partnerships can lower costs through shared funding and negotiated pricing, such as rebate programs, bulk purchasing, and joint funding for community hearing centers.[2,29,36]
Teleaudiology expansion	• Limited broadband access in rural areas and digital literacy barriers among older adults reduce teleaudiology adoption.[20,31,32]	• Federal broadband grants to improve connectivity[2,32] • Community-based digital literacy programs for older adults[2,32] • User-friendly interfaces to enhance accessibility. [2,32] • Enhancing these factors will bolster successful models such as the VA hearing care program, with the potential for these improvements to extend to other insurance delivery systems.[2,31,32]
OTC hearing aid regulation	• Enforcement costs can pose a substantial financial burden.[35,36] • Lack of consumer confidence in the efficacy and safety of OTC hearing aids remains a barrier.[21,34,35]	• Launch campaigns using standardized educational materials to deliver clear, evidence-based information.[2,35] • Establish programs to guide consumers in selecting and effectively using their hearing devices.[2,35] • Implement independent product testing and clearly defined performance benchmarks to create standardized compliance criteria.[2,35] • Leverage external verification to monitor adherence and reduce resource-intensive enforcement activities.[2,35]
Private insurance reform	• Insurers may resist expanding coverage because of cost concerns and financial risk.[2,23]	• Urge insurers to standardize hearing aid benefits using evidence-based guidelines to ensure consistent coverage.[2,23] • Implement risk-sharing agreements between insurers and the government that tie financial responsibility to specific patient outcomes and cost metrics, promoting sustainable coverage availability.[2,23,33]
Artificial intelligence–driven, technology enabled framework	• Data privacy and security risks with health and claims data • Algorithmic bias and inequities in predictions • Technology interoperability and reliability • Provider resistance and workflow disruption.	• Deidentification, federated learning, blockchain audit trails • Diverse data sets, bias audits, recalibration with outcome feedback • Standardized data formats, phased rollouts, certification • Codesign with clinicians and offer efficiency incentives

Note. FMAP = Federal Medical Assistance Percentage; OTC = over the counter; VA = Veterans Affairs.

LIMITATIONS

There are certain limitations to this article. It is an analytic essay rather than a systematic review, and as such it draws from an unstructured review of peer-reviewed publications, policy analyses, and regulatory and legislative documents supplemented by targeted consultation of agency and organizational resources. This approach emphasizes breadth and policy relevance but does not follow a protocol-based systematic process, so some emerging studies or reports may not have been captured. The synthesis reflects developments through the first half of 2025, and, given the rapidly evolving policy landscape, periodic reassessment will be needed. Together, these considerations provide a context for the conclusions drawn and the priorities for future research.

CONCLUSIONS

Hearing loss among older adults remains widespread and undertreated, impairing social connections and cognitive health and driving avoidable health care costs.[3–5,8] Despite policy progress, coverage through Medicare, Medicaid, VA, and private insurers is fragmented and often inadequate, limiting affordable care.[16–19] Closing these gaps requires integrating hearing health into mainstream policies with strengthened financing, workforce development, and outreach.[2,13,34,36] System resilience, informed consumers, and equitable access are vital for sustained improvement.[2,35,36] Recent federal approval of OTC devices and CMS efforts to expand audiology access demonstrate promising momentum.[2,6,13,32,35,36] Building on this progress, payment reforms and digital health innovations could help better align incentives.

Looking forward, researchers, economists, and policymakers should collaborate on pilot initiatives, including bundled payment schemes, risk-sharing arrangements, and investments in digital health infrastructure, to identify effective approaches and guide reform. Future research should also update and expand the current evidence base by generating real-world data on the feasibility and scalability of technology-enabled hearing care models, with an emphasis on cost-effectiveness, workforce integration, and equity across diverse populations. These steps will help foster a hearing health care system that is accessible, affordable, and resilient. AJPH

ABOUT THE AUTHORS

The authors are with the Department of Geriatric Medicine, Yale University, New Haven, CT. Richard Marottoli and Andrew B. Cohen are also with the Yale Pepper Center for Older Adults and the Department of Veterans Affairs at West Haven, West Haven, CT.

CORRESPONDENCE

Correspondence should be sent to Meghana Rajashekara Swamy, MD, MPH, MS, Yale University, Department of Geriatric Medicine, 367 Cedar St, Harkness A, Suite 411, New Haven, CT 06510 (e-mail: meghana.rajashekara@gmail.com). Reprints can be ordered at https://www.ajph.org by clicking the "Reprints" link.

PUBLICATION INFORMATION

Full Citation: Swamy MR, Marottoli R, Cohen AB. Bridging the hearing divide: policy solutions for aging Americans. *Am J Public Health*. 2026; 116(3):387–396.

Acceptance Date: September 19, 2025

DOI: https://doi.org/10.2105/AJPH.2025.308298

ORCID iDs:

Meghana Rajashekara Swamy https://orcid.org/0000-0001-8288-2454

Andrew B. Cohen https://orcid.org/0000-0001-9161-8436

CONTRIBUTORS

M. R. Swamy served as first author and made substantial contributions to the study's conception and design; led data acquisition, analysis, and interpretation; drafted the article; and coordinated revisions. R. Marottoli contributed to the design of the study and provided critical revisions for important intellectual content. A. B. Cohen served as senior author, contributing to data interpretation and assisting with drafting and revising the article for intellectual content and overall direction.

ACKNOWLEDGMENTS

Funding for this research was provided by the National Institutes of Health under grant 5T32AG019134. This T32 training grant supports postdoctoral trainees in aging-related research, contributing to the academic and professional development of Meghana Rajashekara Swamy; although not specifically allocated to this project, the grant facilitated the time and effort dedicated to the work. Additional support was provided by the Yale Claude D. Pepper Older Americans Independence Center (grant P30AG21342), funded by the National Institute on Aging; although it did not directly fund the project, this grant supported the time and effort of Richard Marottoli and Andrew B. Cohen.

Note. The institutional support and academic environment provided by Yale University, the Yale Pepper Center for Older Adults, and the Department of Veterans Affairs at West Haven were instrumental in facilitating this work. The authors acknowledge that their institutional affiliations supported the research process; however, the views expressed in this article are solely those of the authors and do not necessarily represent the official policies or positions of the Department of Geriatric Medicine at Yale University, the Department of Veterans Affairs at West Haven, or the Yale Pepper Center for Older Adults.

CONFLICTS OF INTEREST

The authors declare no conflicts of interest.

HUMAN PARTICIPANT PROTECTION

This study did not require institutional review board approval because only publicly available data were used.

REFERENCES

1. Goman AM, Lin FR. Prevalence of hearing loss by severity in the United States. *Am J Public Health.* 2016;106(10):1820–1822. https://doi.org/10.2105/AJPH.2016.303299
2. National Academies of Sciences, Engineering, and Medicine. *Hearing Health Care for Adults: Priorities for Improving Access and Affordability.* Washington, DC: National Academies Press; 2016.
3. Lin FR, Yaffe K, Xia J, et al. Hearing loss and cognitive decline in older adults. *JAMA Intern Med.* 2013;173(4):293–299. https://doi.org/10.1001/jamainternmed.2013.1868
4. Lin FR, Ferrucci L. Hearing loss and falls among older adults in the United States. *Arch Intern Med.* 2012;172(4):369–371. https://doi.org/10.1001/archinternmed.2011.728
5. Choi J, Kim H, Lee J, et al. The association between hearing loss and depression in older adults: a systematic review and meta-analysis. *J Affect Disord.* 2020;265:546–556. https://doi.org/10.1016/j.jad.2020.01.032
6. US Food and Drug Administration. Medical devices; ear, nose, and throat devices; establishing over-the-counter hearing aids; final rule. *Fed Regist.* 2022;87(159):50698–50778.
7. US Census Bureau. *Demographic Turning Points for the United States: Population Projections for 2020 to 2060.* Washington, DC: US Department of Commerce; 2020.
8. Livingston G, Huntley J, Liu KY, et al. Dementia prevention, intervention, and care: 2024 report of the Lancet Standing Commission. *Lancet.* 2024;404(10452):572–628. https://doi.org/10.1016/S0140-6736(24)01296-0
9. Lin FR, Pike JR, Albert MS, et al. Hearing intervention versus health education control to reduce cognitive decline in older adults with hearing loss: the Aging and Cognitive Health Evaluation in Elders randomized trial. *Lancet.* 2023;402(10404):786–797. Published online July 18, 2023. https://doi.org/10.1016/S0140-6736(23)01406-X
10. Butler SM. Caring for an aging US population—the good news and the bad news. *JAMA Health Forum.* 2024;5(5):e241893. https://doi.org/10.1001/jamahealthforum.2024.1893

11. Lin HW, Mahboubi H, Bhattacharyya N. Self-reported hearing difficulty and risk of accidental injury in US adults, 2007 to 2015. *JAMA Otolaryngol Head Neck Surg.* 2018;144(5):413–417. https://doi.org/10.1001/jamaoto.2018.0039

12. Kamil RJ, Lin FR. The effects of hearing impairment in older adults on communication partners: a systematic review. *J Am Acad Audiol.* 2015;26(2):155–182. https://doi.org/10.3766/jaaa.26.2.6

13. World Health Organization. Global costs of unaddressed hearing loss and cost-effectiveness of interventions. Available at: https://apps.who.int/iris/bitstream/10665/254659/1/9789241512046-eng.pdf. Accessed January 23, 2025.

14. Agrawal Y, Platz EA, Niparko JK. Prevalence of hearing loss and differences by demographic characteristics among US adults: data from the National Health and Nutrition Examination Survey, 1999–2004. *Arch Intern Med.* 2008;168(14):1522–1530. https://doi.org/10.1001/archinte.168.14.1522

15. Nieman C, Plaat K, Johnston D, et al. Dementia and hearing care disparities: prevalence of proxy-rated hearing loss and hearing aid use in a community-dwelling cohort of diverse older adults with dementia. *Alzheimers Dement.* 2018;14:P1033. https://doi.org/10.1016/j.jalz.2018.06.2813

16. Reed N, Morales EG, Willink A. Trends in hearing aid use among older adults in the United States, 2011–2018. *Innov Aging.* 2020;4(suppl 1):105. https://doi.org/10.1093/geroni/igaa057.346

17. Reed NS, Garcia-Morales EE, Myers C, et al. Prevalence of hearing loss and hearing aid use among US Medicare beneficiaries aged 71 years and older. *JAMA Netw Open.* 2023;6(7):e2326320. https://doi.org/10.1001/jamanetworkopen.2023.26320

18. Centers for Disease Control and Prevention. Percentage of adults aged 45 and over who use hearing aids: United States, 2021. Available at: https://www.cdc.gov/nchs/products/databriefs/db414.html. Accessed January 21, 2025.

19. McCormack A, Fortnum H. Why do people fitted with hearing aids not wear them? *Int J Audiol.* 2013;52(5):360–368. https://doi.org/10.3109/14992027.2013.769066

20. Johnson P, Morales EG, Reed N. Disparities in hearing aid use among those with hearing loss in rural and urban settings. *Laryngoscope Investig Otolaryngol.* 2025;10(2):e70125. https://doi.org/10.1002/lio2.70125

21. Stephenson J. FDA finalizes rule to allow over-the-counter hearing aids. *JAMA Health Forum.* 2022;3(8):e223672. https://doi.org/10.1001/jamahealthforum.2022.3672

22. Centers for Medicare & Medicaid Services. Audiology services: physician fee schedule. Updated Available at: https://www.cms.gov/medicare/payment/fee-schedules/physician/audiology-services. Accessed May 1, 2025.

23. Mahmoudi E, Zazove P, Meade M, et al. Association between hearing aid use and health care use and cost among older adults with hearing loss. *JAMA Otolaryngol Head Neck Surg.* 2018;144(6):498–505. https://doi.org/10.1001/jamaoto.2018.0273

24. McNeal MH. Say what? The Affordable Care Act, Medicare, and hearing aids. *Harv J Legis.* 2016;53(2):621–670.

25. Department of Health Care Services. Hearing aid coverage FAQ. Available at: https://www.dhcs.ca.gov/services/Pages/HearingAidCapFAQ.aspx. Accessed January 22, 2025.

26. Arizona Health Care Cost Containment System. AHCCCS medical policy manual, policy 310-L covered services. Available at: https://www.azahcccs.gov/shared/Downloads/MedicalPolicyManual/300/310-L.pdf. Accessed January 22, 2025.

27. Kaiser Family Foundation. Potential costs and impact of health provisions in the Build Back Better Act. Available at: https://www.kff.org/health-costs/issue-brief/potential-costs-and-impact-of-health-provisions-in-the-build-back-better-act. Accessed January 22, 2025.

28. Medicare.gov. Hearing aid coverage. Available at: https://www.medicare.gov/coverage/hearing-aids. Accessed May 1, 2025.

29. Bessen SY, Garcia-Morales EE, Lin FR, Reed NS. Use of hearing services in traditional Medicare and Medicare Advantage. *JAMA Health Forum.* 2024;5(10):e243619. https://doi.org/10.1001/jamahealthforum.2024.3619

30. Congress.gov. Medicare Hearing Aid Coverage Act of 2021, HR 477 (2021). Available at: https://www.congress.gov/bill/117th-congress/house-bill/1118. Accessed May 1, 2025.

31. Gallagher TJ, Hori K, Choi JS. Access to hearing healthcare and barriers among United States veterans: a survey-based study. *OTO Open.* 2025;9(1):e70055. https://doi.org/10.1002/oto2.70055

32. Jacobs PG, Saunders GH. New opportunities and challenges for teleaudiology within Department of Veterans Affairs. *J Rehabil Res Dev.* 2014;51(5):vii–xii. https://doi.org/10.1682/JRRD.2014.04.0093

33. Jilla AM, Johnson CE, Huntington-Klein N. Hearing aid affordability in the United States. *Disabil Rehabil Assist Technol.* 2023;18(3):246–252. https://doi.org/10.1080/17483107.2020.1822449

34. Borre ED, Johri M, Dubno JR, et al. Potential clinical and economic outcomes of over-the-counter hearing aids in the US. *JAMA Otolaryngol Head Neck Surg.* 2023;149(7):607–614. https://doi.org/10.1001/jamaoto.2023.0949

35. US Food and Drug Administration. OTC hearing aids: what you should know. Available at: https://www.fda.gov/medical-devices/hearing-aids/otc-hearing-aids-what-you-should-know. Accessed May 1, 2025.

36. Blustein J, Weinstein BE. Opening the market for lower cost hearing aids: regulatory change can improve the health of older Americans. *Am J Public Health.* 2016;106(6):1032–1035. https://doi.org/10.2105/ajph.2016.303176

37. Congressional Research Service. Medicaid's Federal Medical Assistance Percentage (FMAP). Available at: https://www.congress.gov/crs-product/R43847. Accessed May 1, 2025.

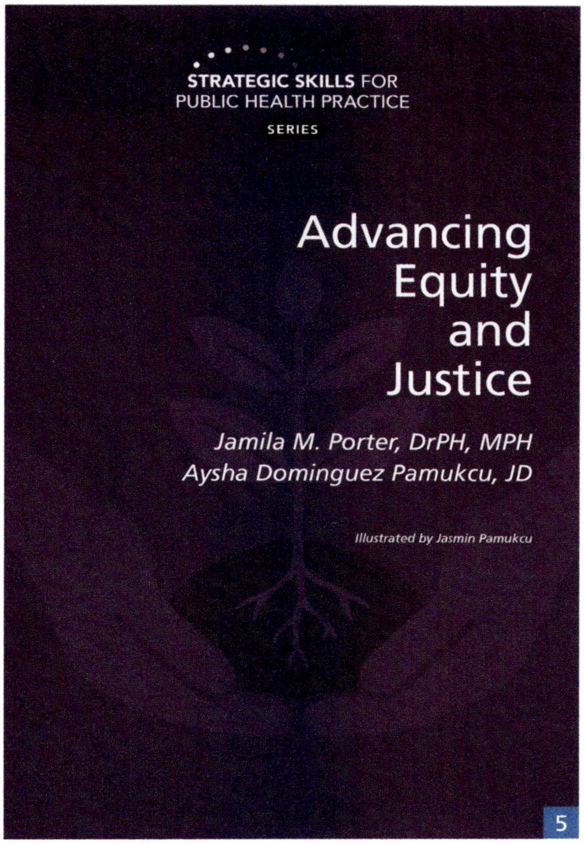

ISBN 978-0-87553-3599, 220 PP., 2026,
SOFTCOVER, PRINT ON DEMAND

Strategic Skills for Public Health Practice: Advancing Equity and Justice

Jamila M. Porter, DrPH, MPH, and Aysha Dominguez Pamukcu, JD

Strategic Skills for Public Health Practice: Advancing Equity and Justice is a call to reimagine public health as a dynamic social movement rooted in community leadership. Grounded in bold vision and practical application, this book confronts the root causes of health inequities — powerful systems that determine how long and how well we live. *Advancing Equity and Justice* challenges practitioners to move beyond limited technical fixes to embrace the moral clarity and collective action necessary to improve health for all.

APHABOOKSTORE.ORG

APHA PRESS

AN IMPRINT OF AMERICAN PUBLIC HEALTH ASSOCIATION